Diet Doodle Diary

I want to be healthier

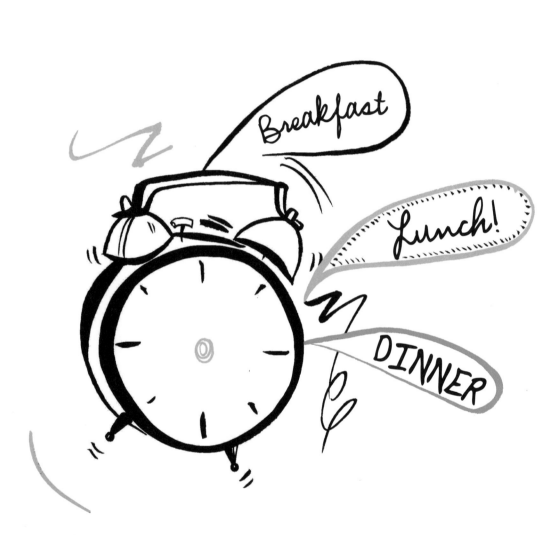

Diet Doodle Diary

In which I record my

Small but SIGNIFICANT slimming TRIUMPHS

Illustrated by
Julie Mackey

PaRragon

Bath · New York · Singapore · Hong Kong · Cologne · Delhi
Melbourne · Amsterdam · Johannesburg · Shenzhen

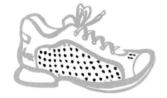

First published by Parragon in 2013

Parragon
Queen Street House
4 Queen Street
Bath BA1 1HE, UK
www.parragon.com

Illustrations by Julie Mackey
Typeset by Waverley Books in Prophecy Script (© Tension Type) and Secret Service Typewriter (© Red Rooster) fonts

Diet Doodle Diary contains real-life tips from genuinely successful dieters—Sandy Fleming, Gill Brown, Susan MacMillan, Sarah Robertson, Jillian Stewart, and Marie Jo McCrossan

ISBN 978-1-78186-827-0
GTIN 5060292801070
Printed in China

Consult your doctor before following any new diet or fitness plans.

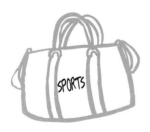

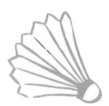

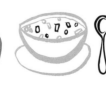

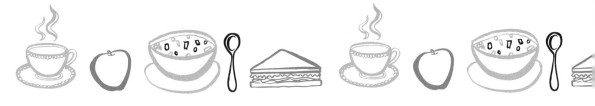

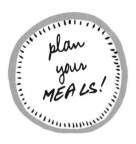

plan
your
MEALS!

The *Diet Doodle Diary* is more than a log book
for your food and exercise.

Write in it, read it, doodle in it, be
inspired—and laugh. Every page has something
to amuse, advise, or make you think.

There are weight-loss secrets from real
dieters who've been there and learned the
hard way. Every page has a tip to make losing
weight easier.

With humorous illustrations by artist Julie
Mackey, this book is the most fun you'll ever
have keeping a weight-loss log!

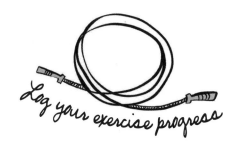

Log your exercise progress

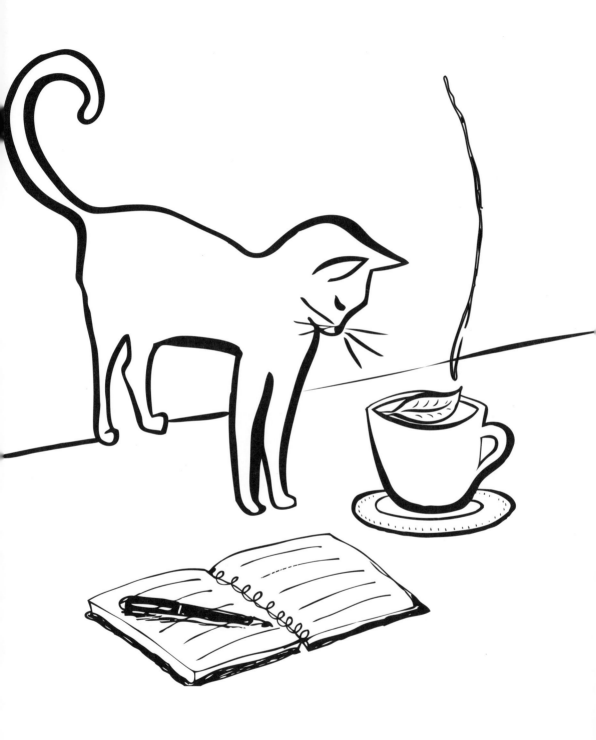

Write

. . . . . .

DRAW

. . . . .

LOG

. . . . .

chart your
PROGRESS

. . . . .

Be inspired

Record Your Measurements

.... neck

chest ....

.... upper arm

waist ....

.... wrist

thigh ....

calf ....

.... ankle

Today's Date:

THE weigh-IN

Starting weight:

Resting heart rate:

TIP: How to find your resting heart rate.

On waking, take your pulse using three fingers. Find the pulse in your wrist or your neck—whichever is easier. Count how many heartbeats you can feel in six seconds. Multiply by ten to find how many beats per minute. Write this number in the box above. Every so often throughout the book you'll have space to record this to see how your fitness is improving.

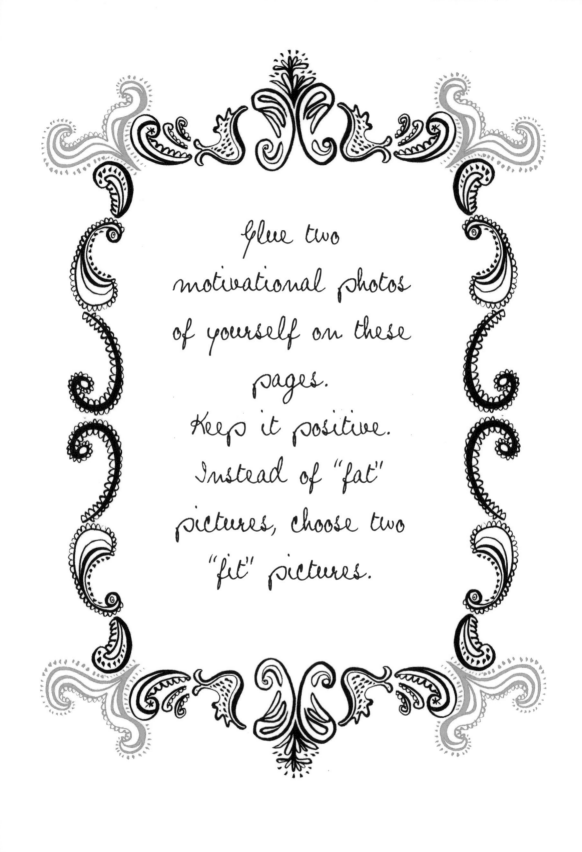

Glue two
motivational photos
of yourself on these
pages.
Keep it positive.
Instead of "fat"
pictures, choose two
"fit" pictures.

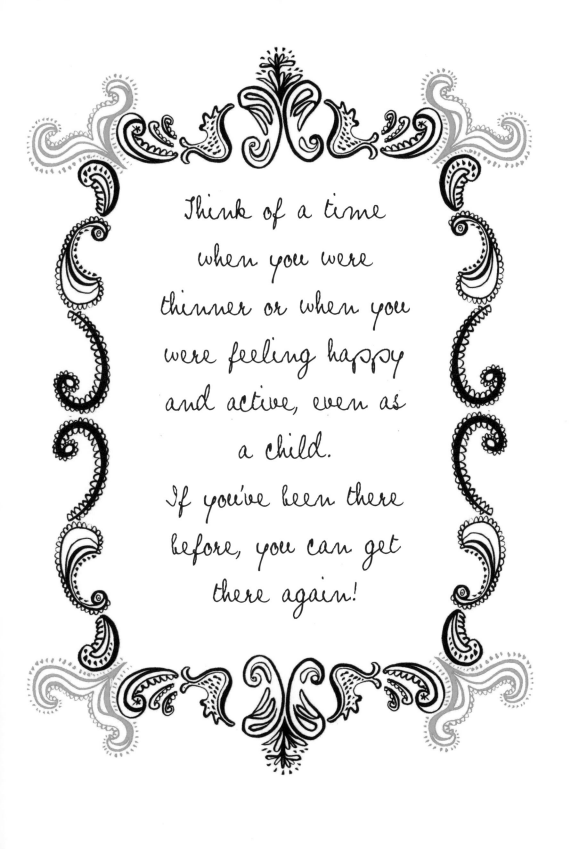

Think of a time
when you were
thinner or when you
were feeling happy
and active, even as
a child.
If you've been there
before, you can get
there again!

"Diet starts Monday?"

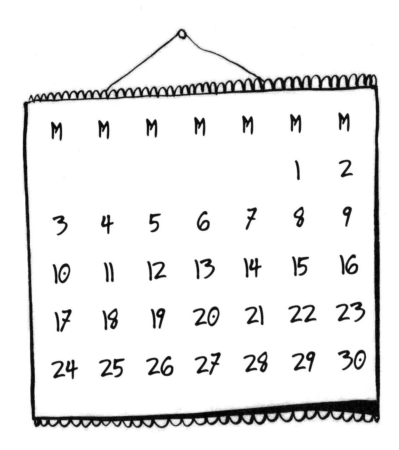

... your healthy eating plan can start any day, don't wait for Monday!

Start by getting rid of all of the junk food in your kitchen.

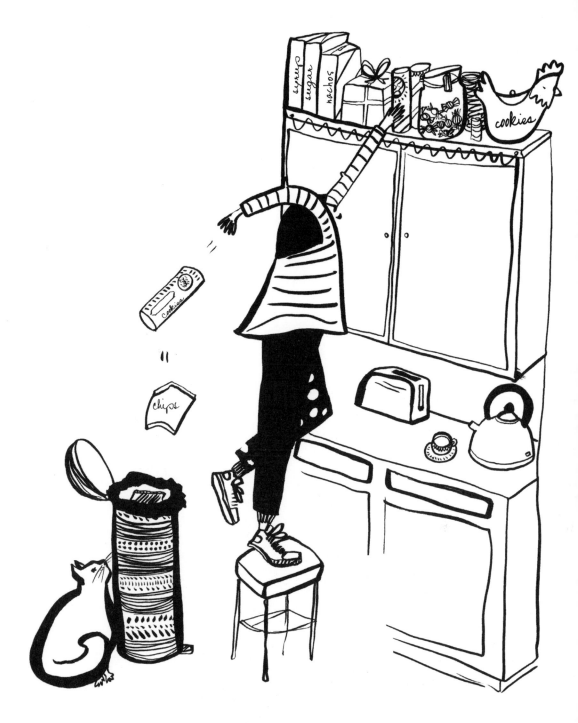

Don't think of it as wasteful. It was trash even when you bought it!

Start keeping a food diary today.

You'll find it helpful to write down everything that you eat.

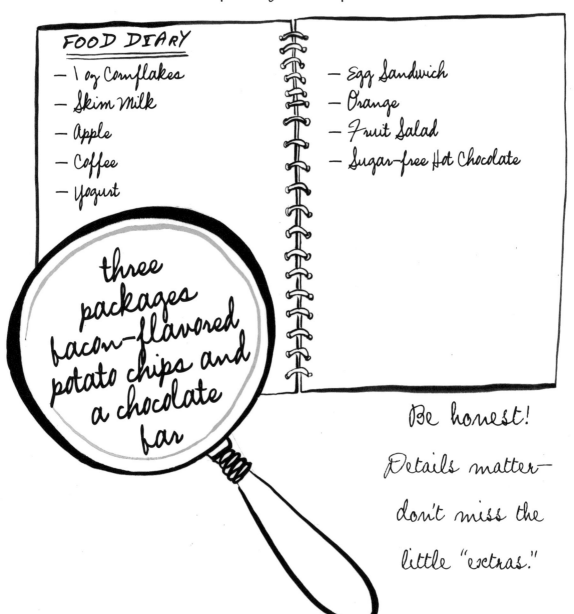

FOOD DIARY

— 1 oz Cornflakes
— Skim Milk
— Apple
— Coffee
— Yogurt

— Egg Sandwich
— Orange
— Fruit Salad
— Sugar-free Hot Chocolate

three packages bacon-flavored potato chips and a chocolate bar

Be honest! Details matter — don't miss the little "extras."

what did you eat

WEEK
1

today?

Monday

Tuesday

Wednesday

Thursday

Friday

Saturday

Sunday

Start keeping an exercise log today.

Rest days and stretch days count too. Make a record of them.

Week 1

| Monday | Tuesday |

| Wednesday | Thursday | Friday |

| Saturday | Sunday |

THE weigh-IN

WEIGHT :

WAIST :

HEART RATE :

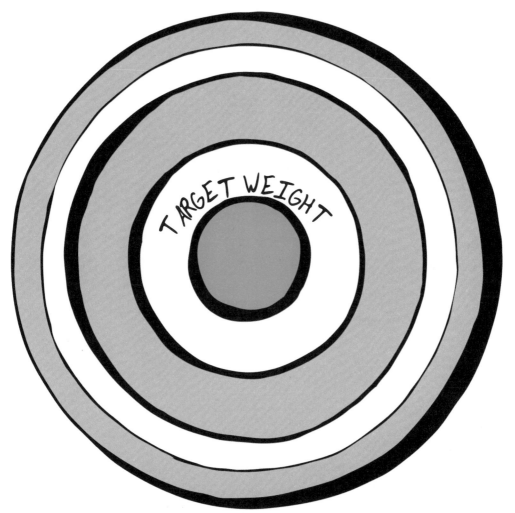

TARGET WEIGHT

Set a target weight you'd like to reach and write it here. Don't make it time-sensitive. Visualize yourself at that weight.

WHAT

ARE

YOUR

FITNESS

goals?

Circle

any of the ones you like

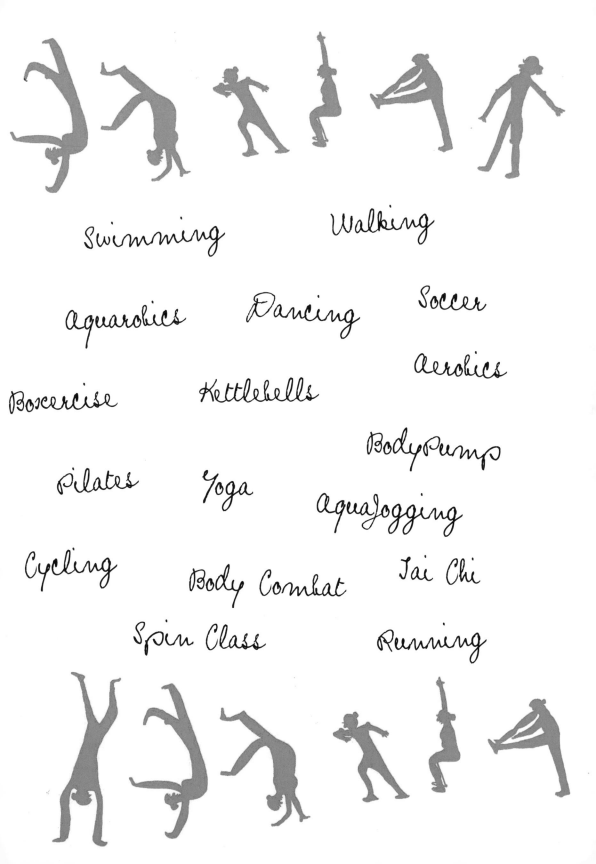

Swimming

Walking

Aquarobics

Dancing

Soccer

Aerobics

Boxercise

Kettlebells

BodyPump

Pilates

Yoga

AquaJogging

Cycling

Body Combat

Tai Chi

Spin Class

Running

Monday

Tuesday

Wednesday

Thursday

Friday

Food
Diary

Saturday

Sunday

WEEK
2

EXERCISE LOG
WEEK 2

Monday

Tuesday

Wednesday

Thursday

Friday

THE weigh-IN

WEIGHT : _____

WAIST : _____

HEART

RATE : _____

Saturday

Sunday

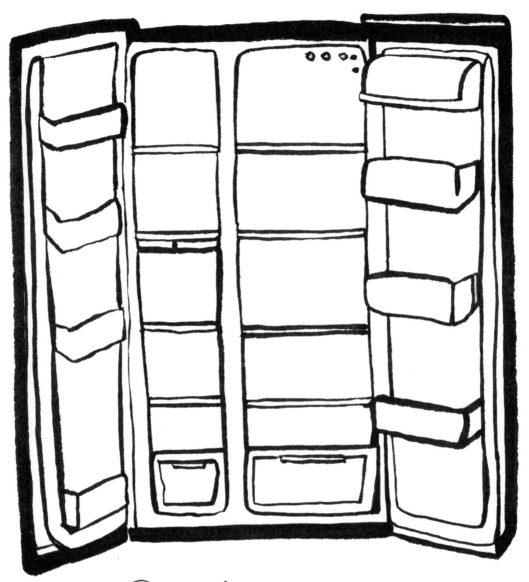

Draw the contents of
your refrigerator as it
looks now—be honest
about it!

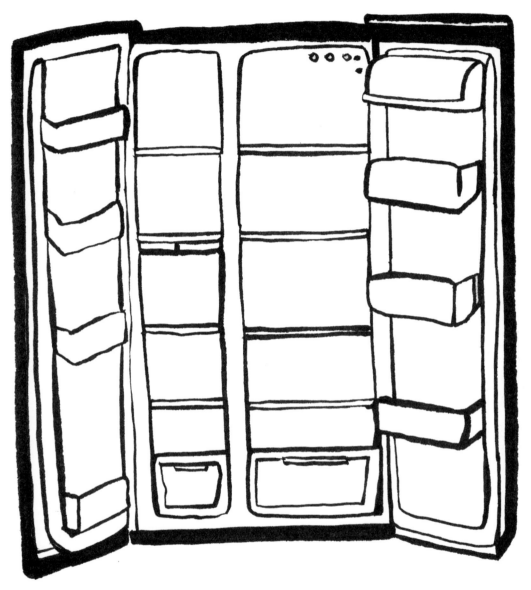

Draw the contents of your refrigerator as it is going to look once you've been shopping for healthy foods.

"By failing to prepare, you are preparing to fail."
-Benjamin Franklin

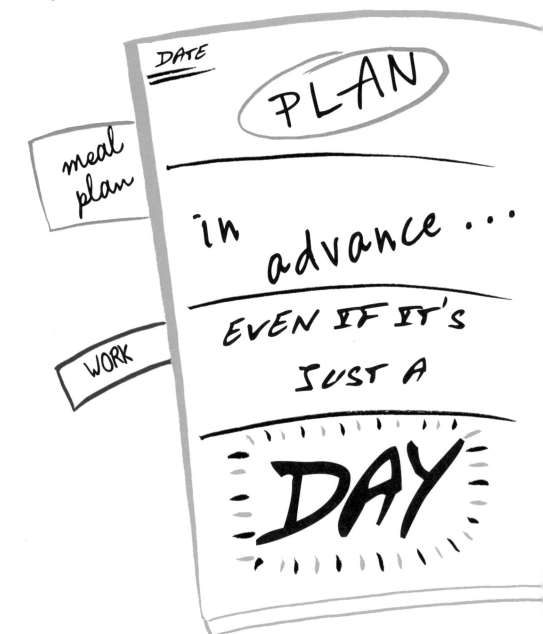

If you
plan ahead

DATE

You will be LESS

likely to...

STRAY from IT!

SHOPPING LIST

exercise plan

Laundry

SOCIAL LIFE!

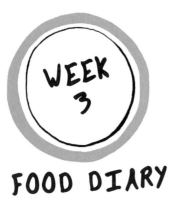

WEEK
3

FOOD DIARY

Monday

Tuesday

Wednesday

Thursday

Friday

Saturday

Sunday

EXERCISE LOG
WEEK 3

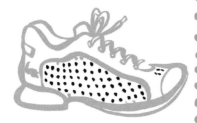

Monday

Tuesday

Wednesday

Thursday

Friday

Saturday

Sunday

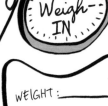

THE Weigh-IN

WEIGHT : _____

WAIST : _____

HEART RATE : _____

REMEMBER: Record your rest and stretch days too.

How do you feel ?

Choose descriptive words and write them
in the thought bubbles. We'll do this again later.

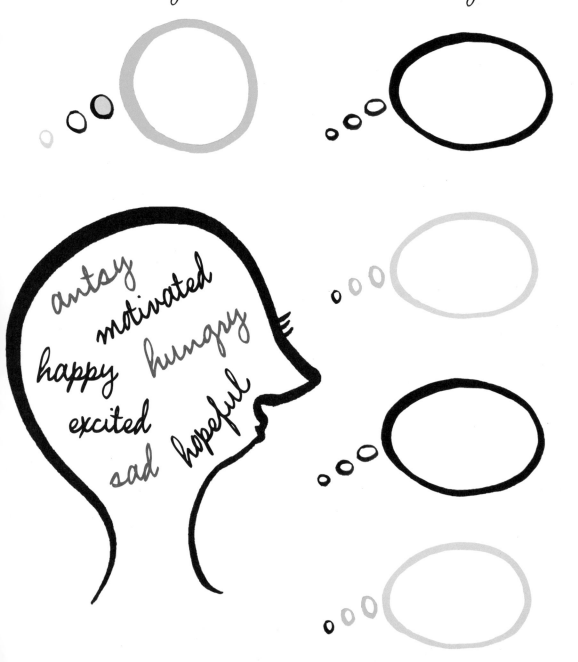

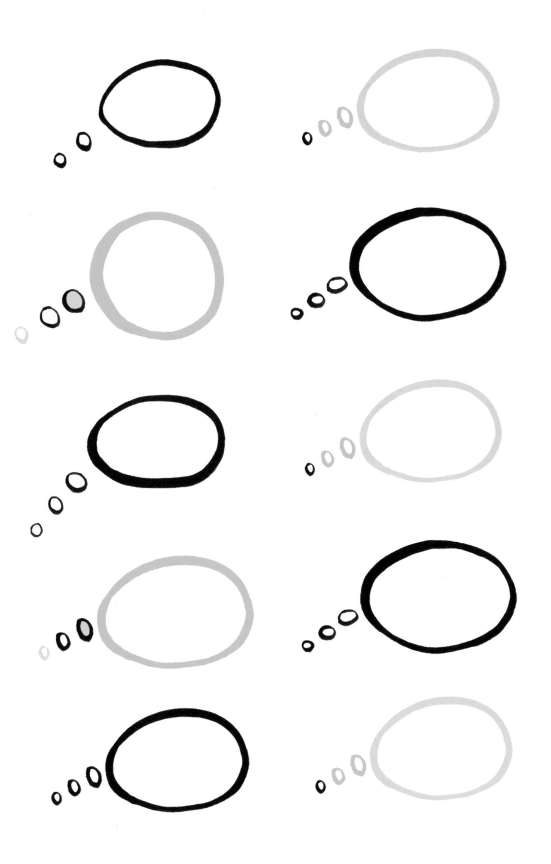

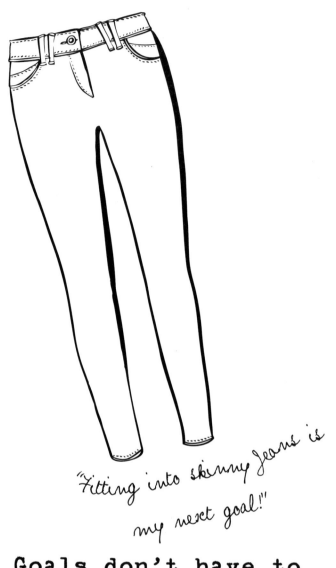

"Fitting into skinny Jeans is my next goal!"

Goals don't have to be about the number on the scales.

My Goals

Write down what your long-term goals are (we'll revisit them later and see how many you've achieved).

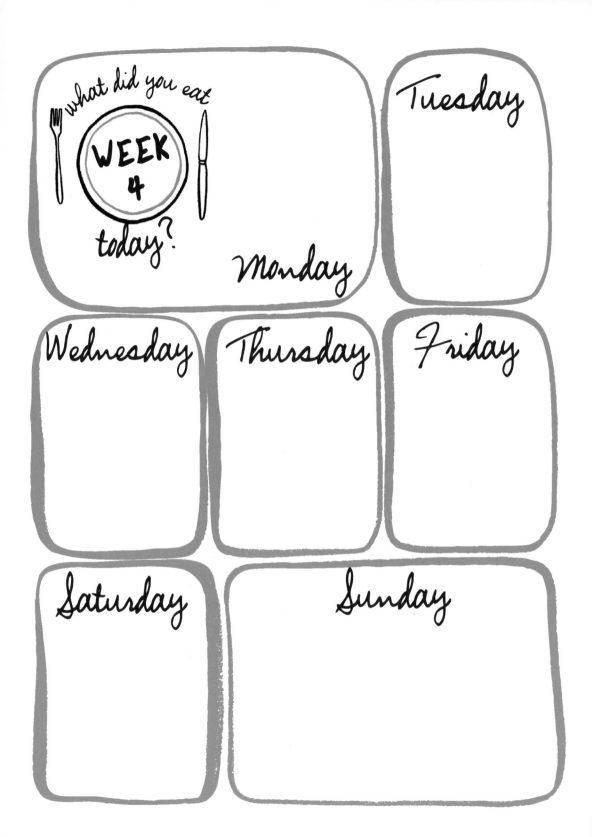

what did you eat

WEEK 4

today?

Monday

Tuesday

Wednesday

Thursday

Friday

Saturday

Sunday

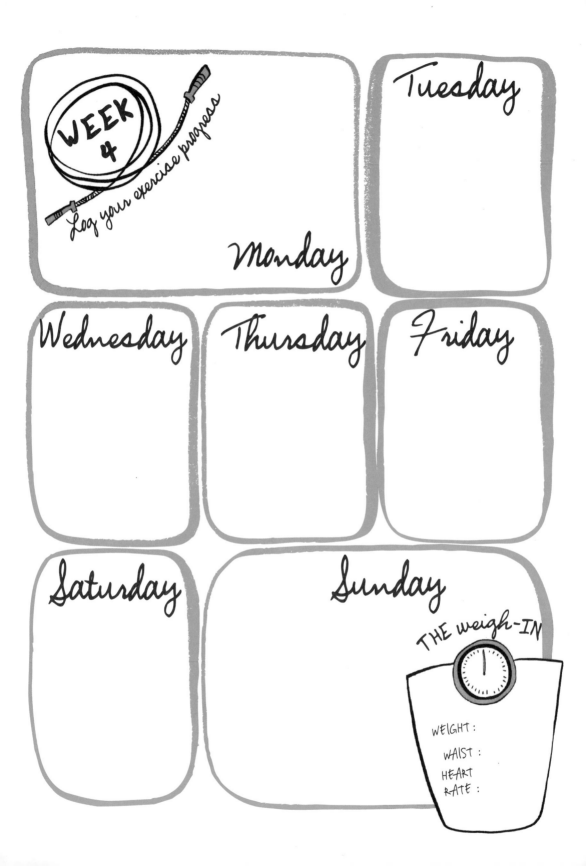

WEEK 4

Log your exercise progress

Monday

Tuesday

Wednesday

Thursday

Friday

Saturday

Sunday

THE weigh-IN

WEIGHT :

WAIST :

HEART
RATE :

THOSE SKINNY JEANS

THEY FIT!

ALMOST!

NEARLY, KEEP GOING!

I CAN DO THIS!

LONG WAY TO GO YET!

Skinny Jeans, or the perfect little dress—too tight and still with the tags on. We've all got something like that in the closet! Well, you said you'd "slim into it," so use it as a goal. On the opposite page, shade how far you've come in your quest to fit into that impulse buy.

Then post your picture here when it fits!

Monday

Tuesday

Wednesday

Thursday

Friday

Saturday

Sunday

WEEK 5

FOOD DIARY

EXERCISE LOG
WEEK 5

Monday

Tuesday

Wednesday

Thursday

Friday

Saturday

Sunday

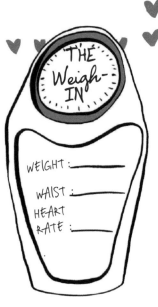

THE Weigh-IN

WEIGHT : _____

WAIST : _____

HEART RATE : _____

Be kind to yourself. Don't say things to yourself that you would never dream of saying to anyone else.

Draw or
write ten things
you like about
yourself
inside the hearts.

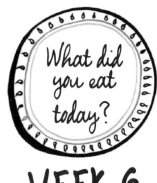

What did you eat today?

WEEK 6

Monday

Tuesday

Wednesday

Thursday

Friday

Saturday

Sunday

Do **YOUR** best

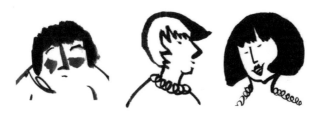

Don't compare yourself with others

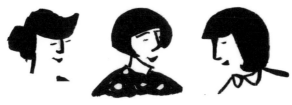

Don't aim for perfection

Be the best that **YOU** can be!

Track Your Progress ...

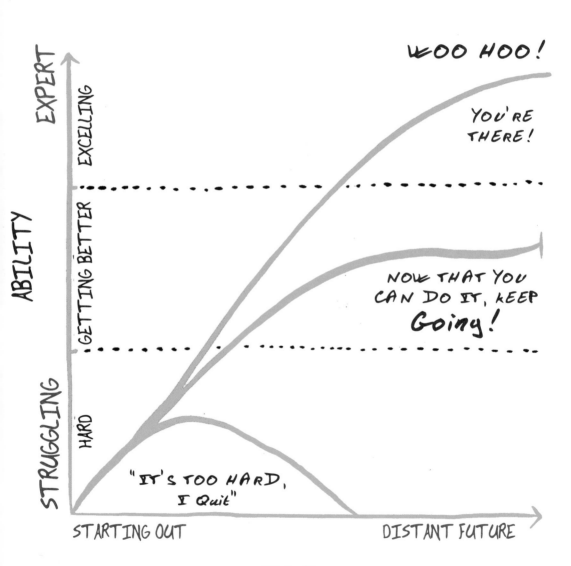

Let's see the line on the
graph go up and up as your
weight comes down and down.

WEIGHT LOSS IN POUNDS

105
100
95
90
85
80
75
70
65
60
55
50
45
40
35
30
25
20
15
10
5

2 4 6 8 10 12 14 16 18 20 22 24 24 26 28 30

WEEKS

Week 6

Log your exercise progress

Monday

Tuesday

Wednesday

Thursday

Friday

Saturday

Sunday

THE weigh-IN

WEIGHT :

WAIST :

HEART RATE :

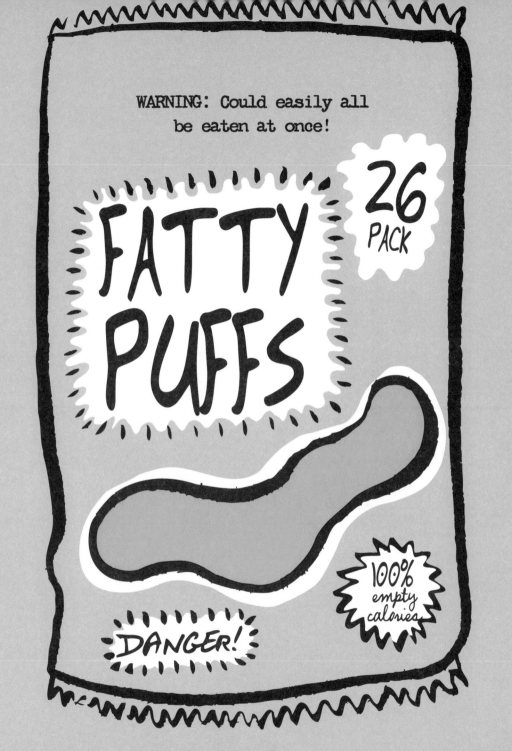

Don't buy multipacks of your favorite snacks or candies, even if they are "on sale."

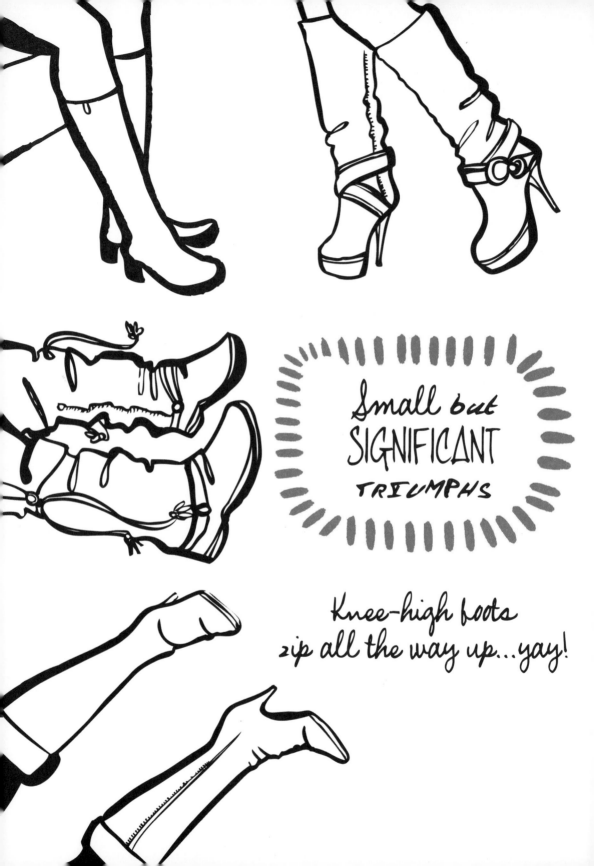

Small but SIGNIFICANT TRIUMPHS

Knee-high boots
zip all the way up...yay!

Monday

Tuesday

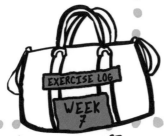

Wednesday

Thursday

Friday

Saturday

Sunday

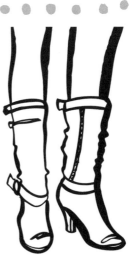

"Whatever I wear today, the boots are going on!"

Have tea or coffee, fruits, and cereal for breakfast.

Leave home feeling full.

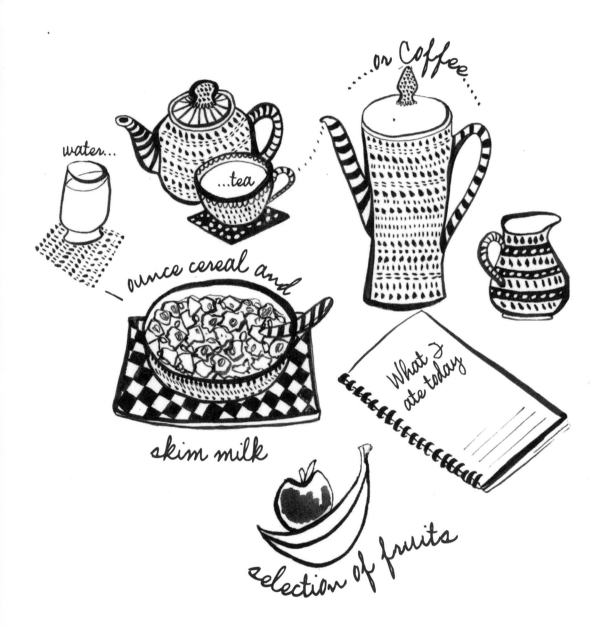

Challenge: make this week's
breakfasts outstanding!

Plan
them
here:

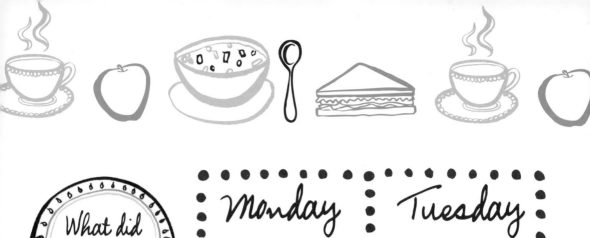

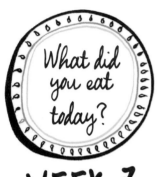

WEEK 7

Monday

Tuesday

Wednesday

Thursday

Friday

Saturday

Sunday

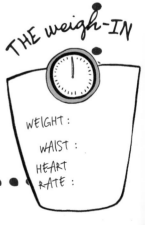

THE weigh-IN

WEIGHT :

WAIST :

HEART RATE :

Don't eat the same thing every day ...
... even if you love it now, you'll get real tired of it.

List your favorite ingredients here ...

Now go find some new recipes and cook from them. Write up new recipes regularly in the spaces provided in this book.

My new recipes

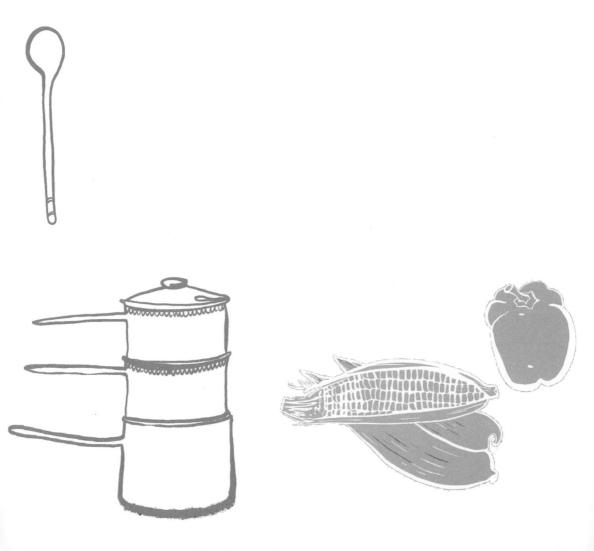

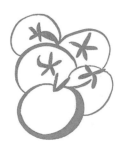

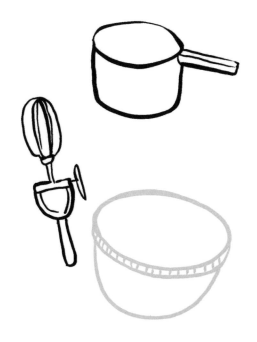

If what you are doing is not WORKING GUESS WHAT? Change what you are DOING!

How do you feel about your progress so far? What little things could you change that might improve your weight loss?

Monday

Tuesday

Wednesday

Thursday

Friday

Saturday

Sunday

EXERCISE
LOG
WEEK 8

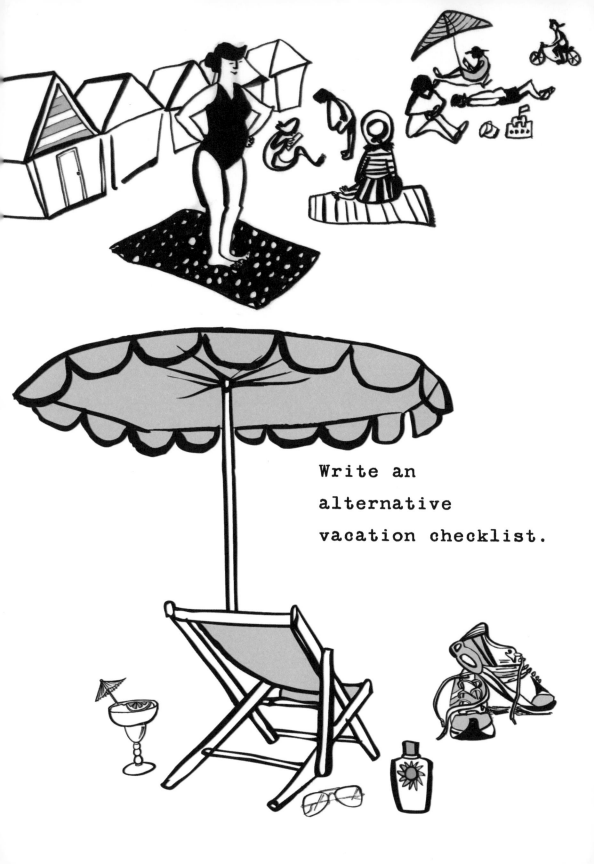

Write an
alternative
vacation checklist.

This checklist isn't going to include a passport and sunscreen, but might include fitting comfortably into an airplane seat and not giving up your healthy eating or your jogging plan just because you are on vacation.

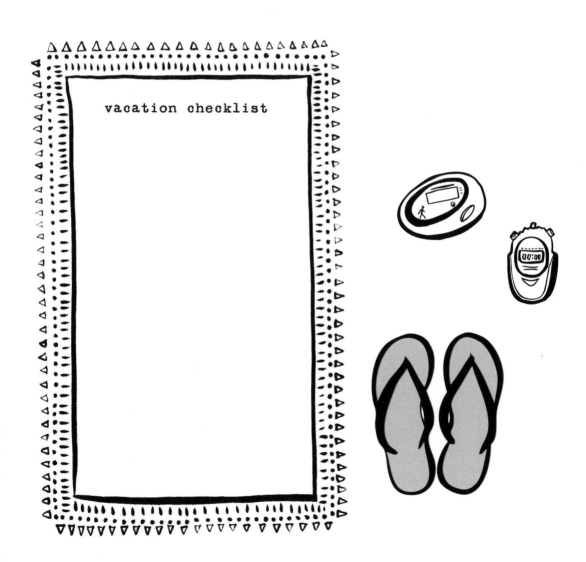

vacation checklist

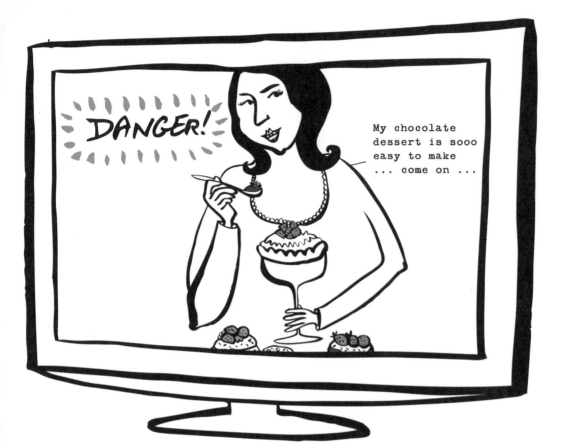

TV cooking shows can seriously threaten your planning.

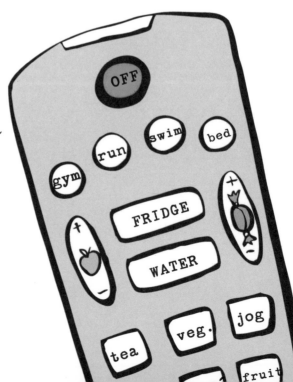

WHAT DID YOU EAT TODAY?

WEEK 8

Monday	Tuesday
Wednesday	Thursday
Friday	
Saturday	Sunday

THE weigh-IN

WEIGHT :

WAIST :

HEART RATE :

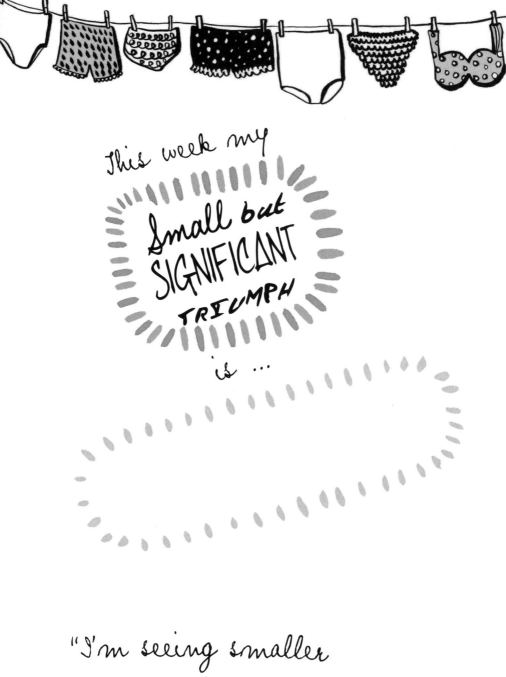

This week my *Small but* SIGNIFICANT TRIUMPH is ...

"I'm seeing smaller panties on my laundry line."

WEEK 9

What did you eat today?

Monday

Tuesday

Wednesday

Thursday

Friday

Saturday

Sunday

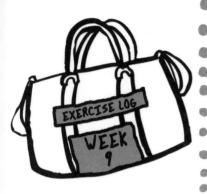

EXERCISE LOG
WEEK 9

Monday

Tuesday

Wednesday

Thursday

Friday

Saturday

Sunday

THE weigh-IN

WEIGHT : _____

WAIST : _____
HEART
RATE : _____

Remember to stretch! And drink water!

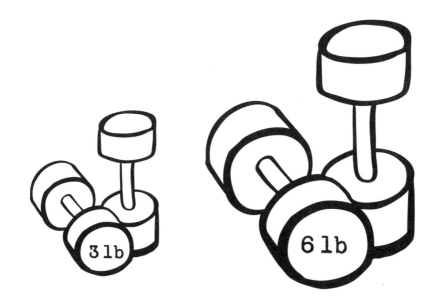

Weights: Day 1   Weights: Day 24

Track your progress.
What seems impossible at the
beginning will get easier
every time you do it.

Does your closet need a clean-out?

This week's challenge: Clean out your too-big clothes, clean out your too-small clothes, clean out your unflattering tent dresses and your worn-out baggy stuff. Coordinate and organize what's left to make the most of your figure.

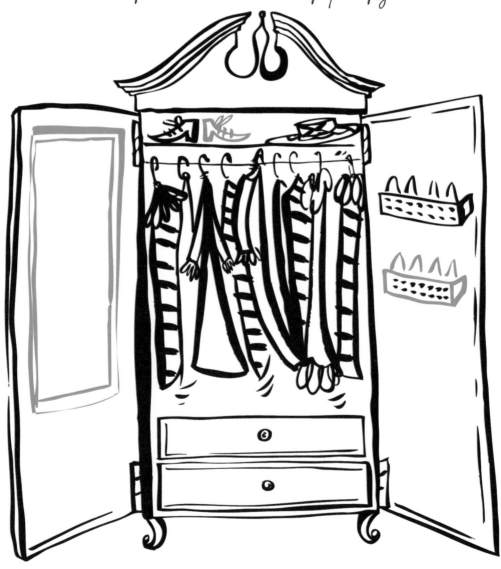

Write or draw here what you need to buy to
complete your current wardrobe:

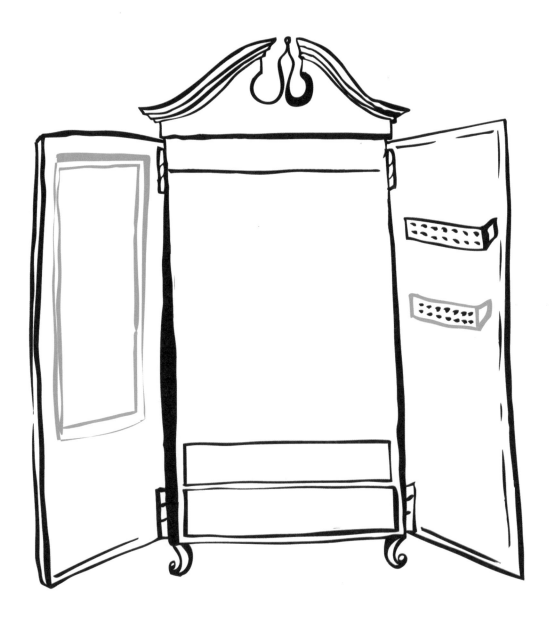

Monday

Tuesday

Wednesday

Thursday

Friday

Saturday

Sunday

What did
you eat
today?

WEEK 10

EXERCISE LOG
WEEK 10

Monday

Tuesday

Wednesday

Thursday

Friday

Saturday

Sunday

THE weigh-IN

WEIGHT : _____

WAIST : _____

HEART
RATE : _____

Exercise is more than "keeping in shape."

Exercise is time for yourself—time to think.

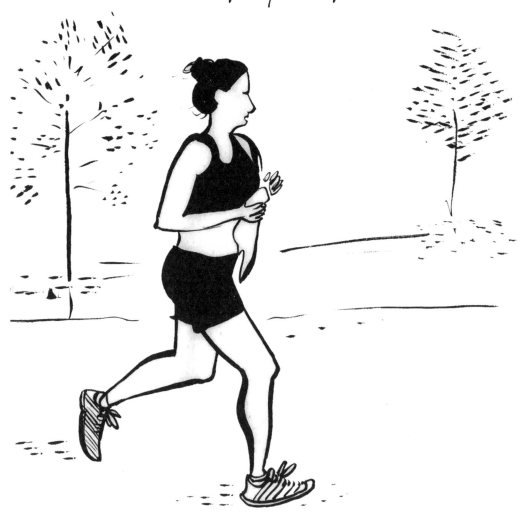

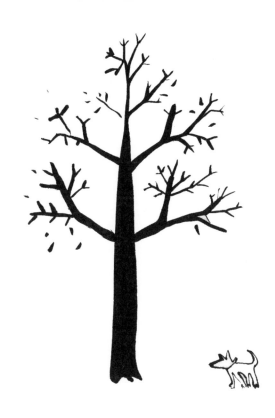

Write down the things you get out of
exercise other than weight loss.

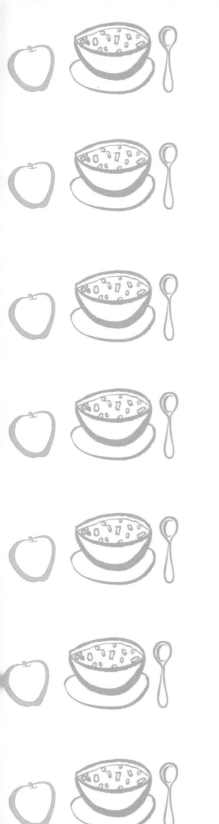

Lunch isn't for wimps.

But don't eat the same thing every day. Write some new lunch ideas here—bagels, wraps, flatbreads, whole grain rice ...

Monday

Tuesday

Wednesday

Thursday

Friday

week 11

Saturday

Sunday

Log your exercise progress

What did you eat today?

WEEK 11

Monday

Tuesday

Wednesday

Thursday

Friday

THE weigh-IN

WEIGHT : _____

WAIST : _____

HEART RATE : _____

Saturday

Sunday

Don't play the lunchtime lottery at the deli ... bring your own lunch.

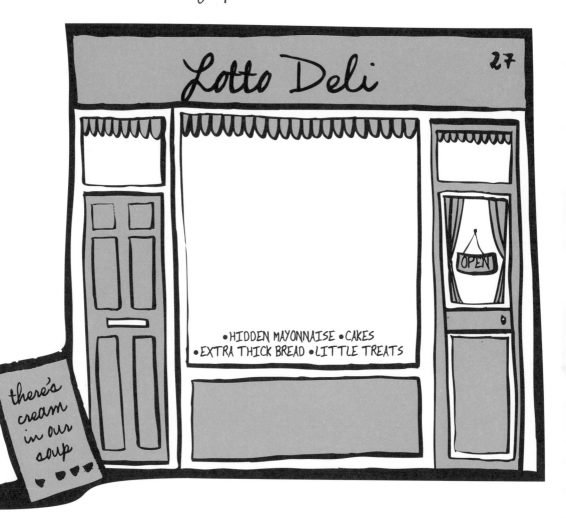

Are you noticing patterns in your food choices?

Challenge!

DON'T MAKE WEIGHT LOSS YOUR ONLY GOAL.

CHALLENGE YOURSELF:

Get more sleep

Be more organized,

precook the week's meals

Learn new recipes

Take a new class

Get a fitness goal

Drink more water

Meet more people

Look more groomed

Bring a brown-bag lunch from home

What could you challenge yourself to do?

Write seven
challenges
here:

Color the
boxes when
they become a
regular thing.

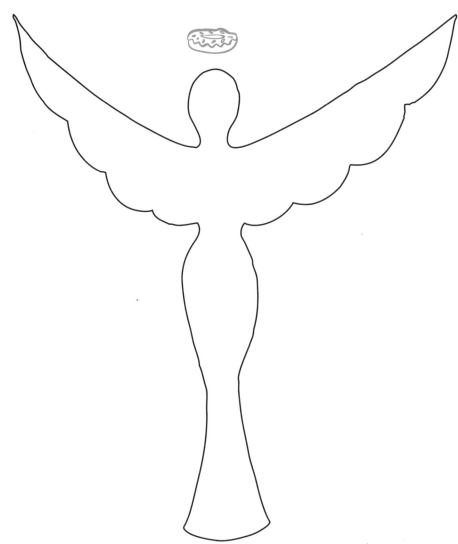

You don't have to be a SAINT,
just be honest with yourself.
You can't eat cookies and candy
EVERY DAY and lose weight.

Log your exercise progress

WEEK 12

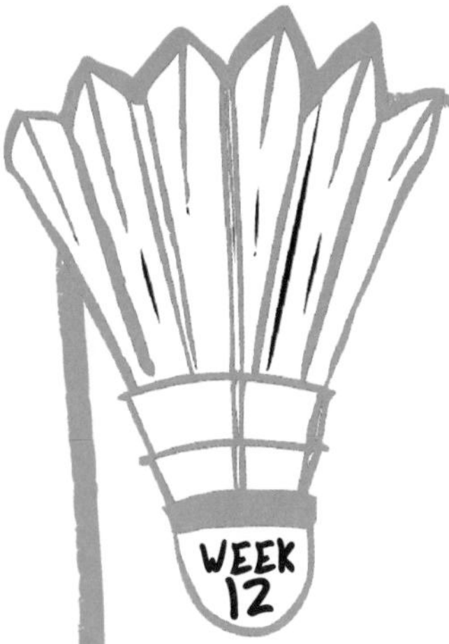

Monday

Tuesday

Wednesday

Thursday

Friday

Saturday

Sunday

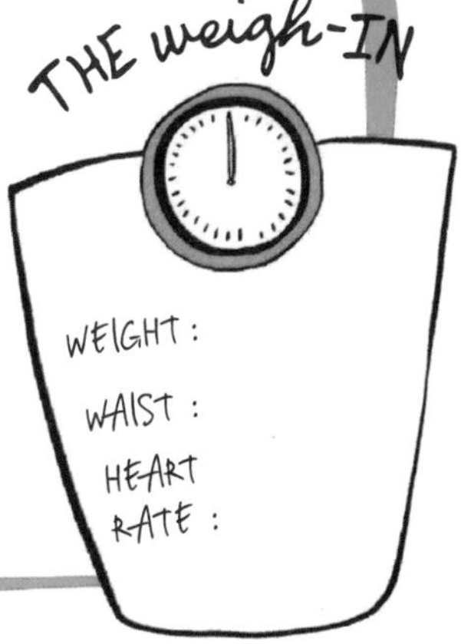

THE weigh-IN
WEIGHT :
WAIST :
HEART RATE :

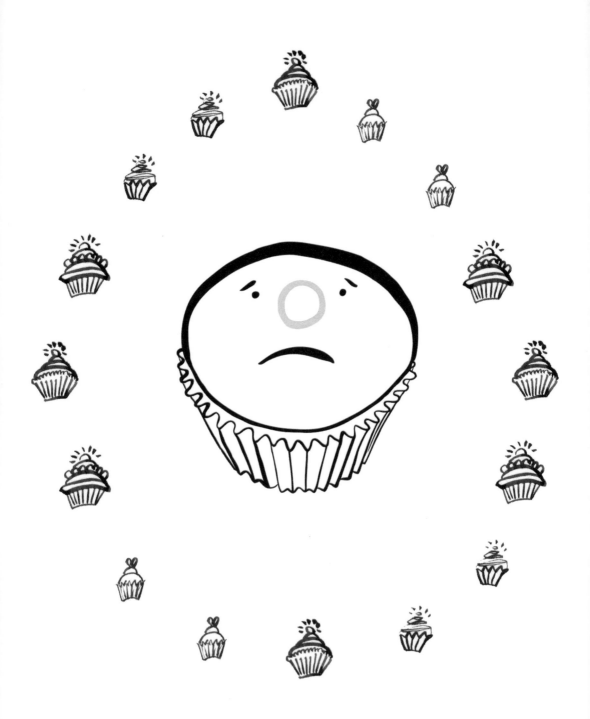

Don't feed your emotions . . . .

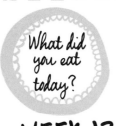

What did you eat today?

WEEK 12

Monday

Tuesday

Wednesday

Thursday

Friday

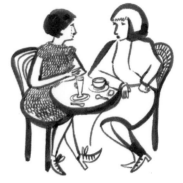

Saturday

Sunday

... deal with problems in other ways, not with food.

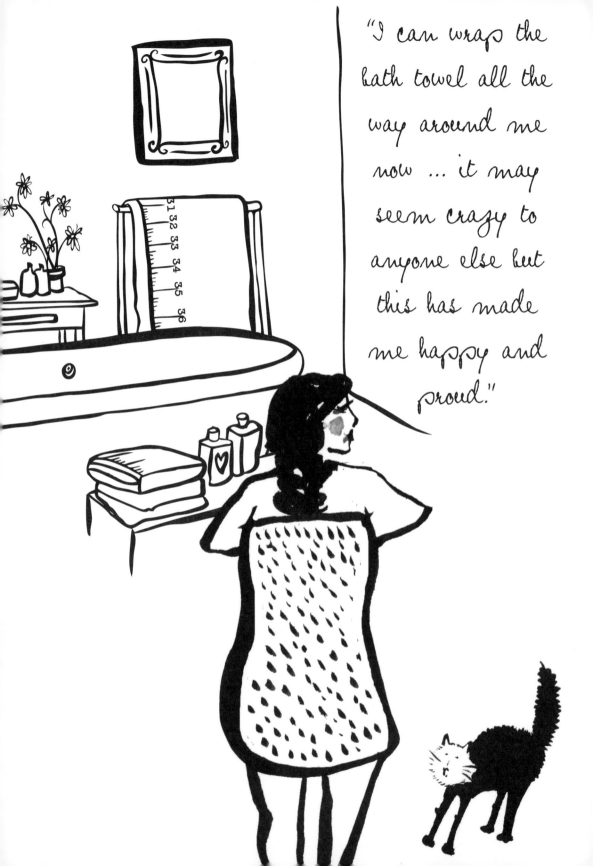

"I can wrap the bath towel all the way around me now ... it may seem crazy to anyone else but this has made me happy and proud."

This week my

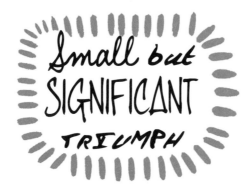

is ...

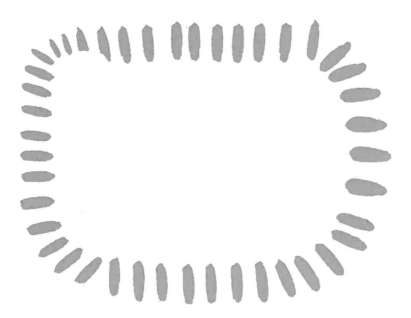

FAST OR Slow?

EAT SLOWER.

Get a timer and make sure
you take at least
20 minutes
to eat every meal.

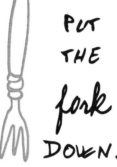

PUT
THE
fork
DOWN.

TICK TOCK.

chew everything real well.

Really TASTE your
food and enjoy it!

Monday

Tuesday

Wednesday

Thursday

Friday

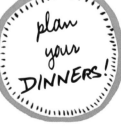
plan
your
DINNERS!

Saturday

Sunday

WEEK 13

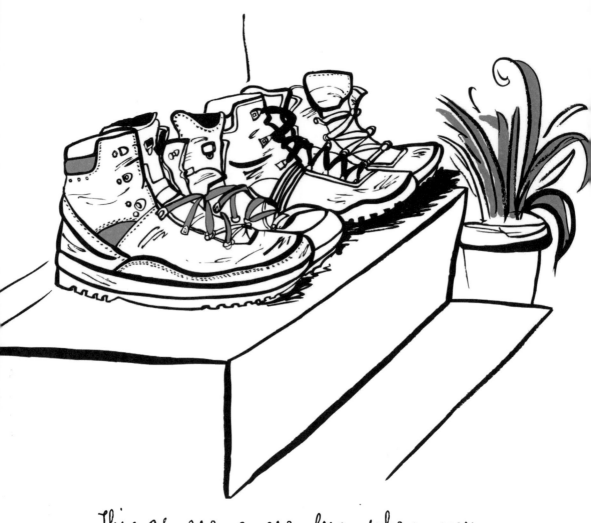

Things are more fun when you do them with someone else—get a friend to join you for exercise.

Monday

Tuesday

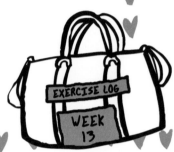

EXERCISE LOG

WEEK 13

Wednesday

Thursday

Friday

Saturday

Sunday

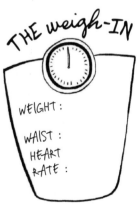

THE weigh-IN

WEIGHT :

WAIST :

HEART
RATE :

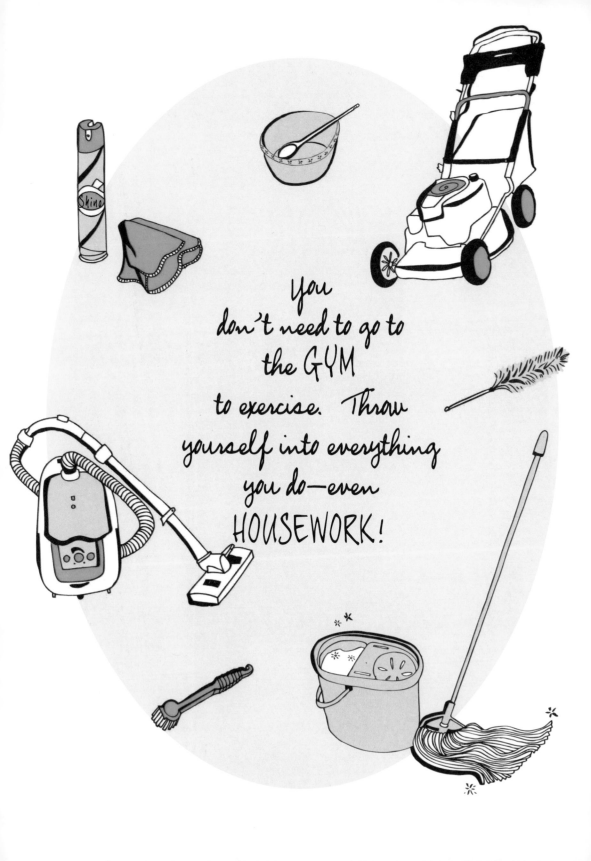

You don't need to go to the GYM to exercise. Throw yourself into everything you do—even HOUSEWORK!

What activities could you do with a little more zing?
Write them here:

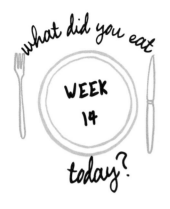

what did you eat

WEEK 14

today?

Monday

Tuesday

Wednesday

Thursday

Friday

Saturday

Sunday

EXERCISE LOG

WEEK 14

Monday

Tuesday

Wednesday

Thursday

Friday

Saturday

Sunday

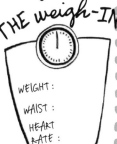

THE weigh-IN

WEIGHT :

WAIST :

HEART RATE :

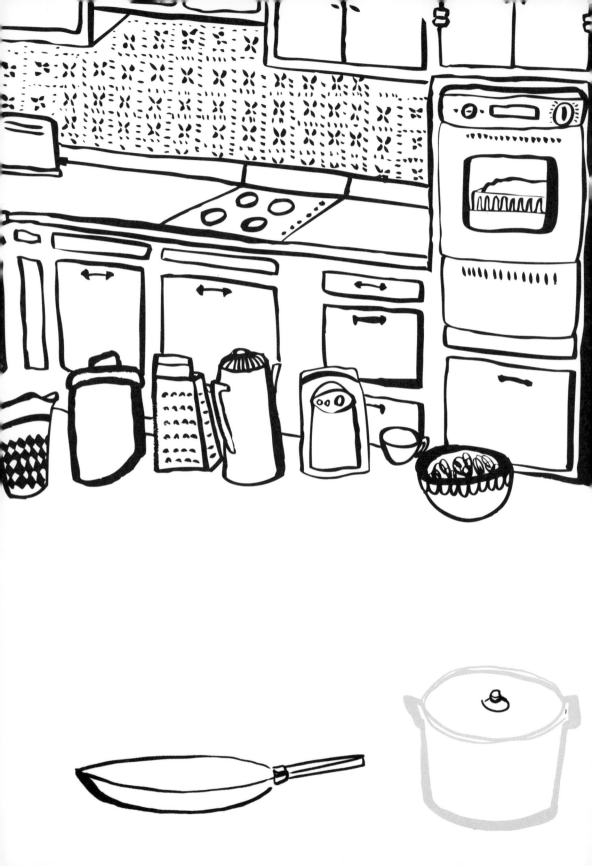

my NEW recipes

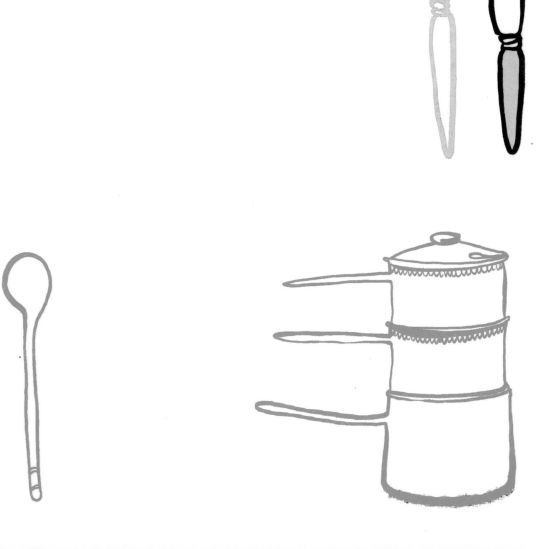

Monday

Tuesday

Wednesday

Thursday

Friday

what did you eat

WEEK 15

today?

Saturday

Sunday

Food before:
spaghetti and wine
and garlic bread

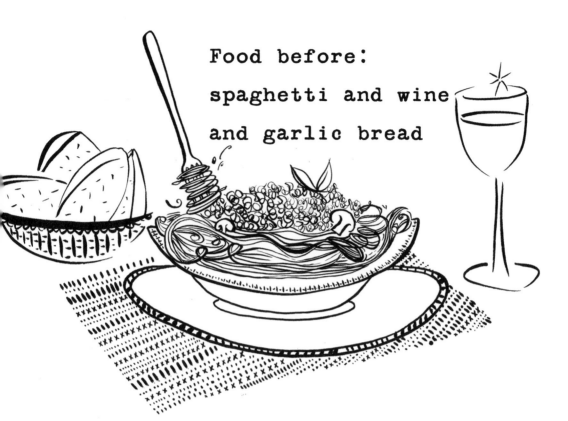

Food now: still
looks good!

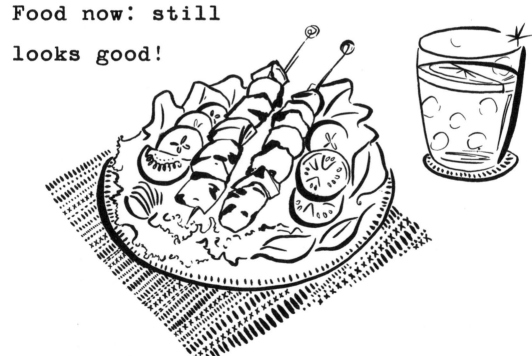

Writing down your
goals makes it
more likely that
you'll strive to
achieve them...

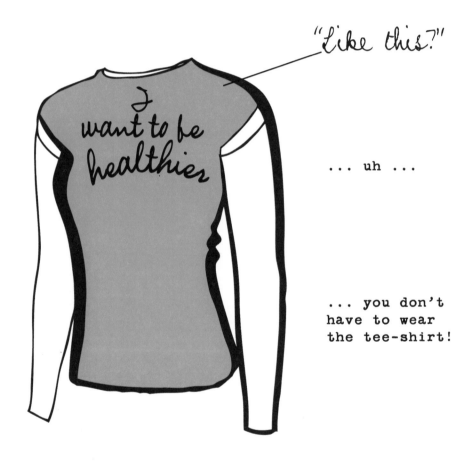

"Like this?"

... uh ...

... you don't
have to wear
the tee-shirt!

Just write them down and keep them in a
place where you'll see them every day.

Log your fitness progress

WEEK 15

Monday

Tuesday

Wednesday

Thursday

Friday

THE Weigh-IN

WEIGHT : _____

WAIST : _____

HEART RATE : _____

Saturday

Sunday

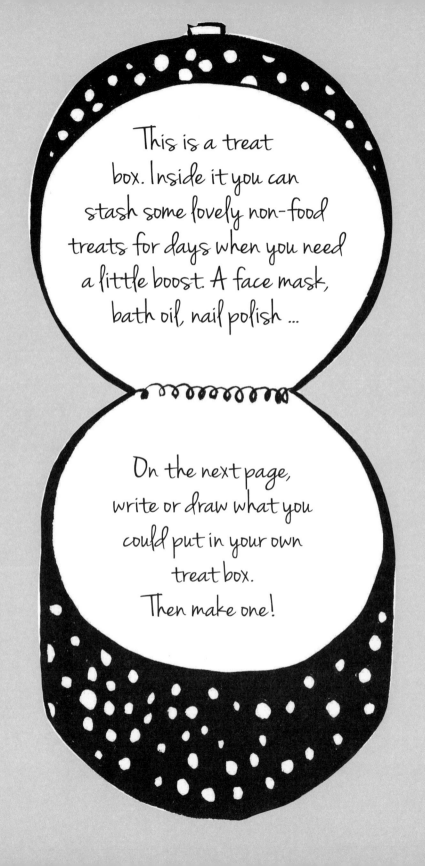

This is a treat box. Inside it you can stash some lovely non-food treats for days when you need a little boost. A face mask, bath oil, nail polish ...

On the next page, write or draw what you could put in your own treat box.
Then make one!

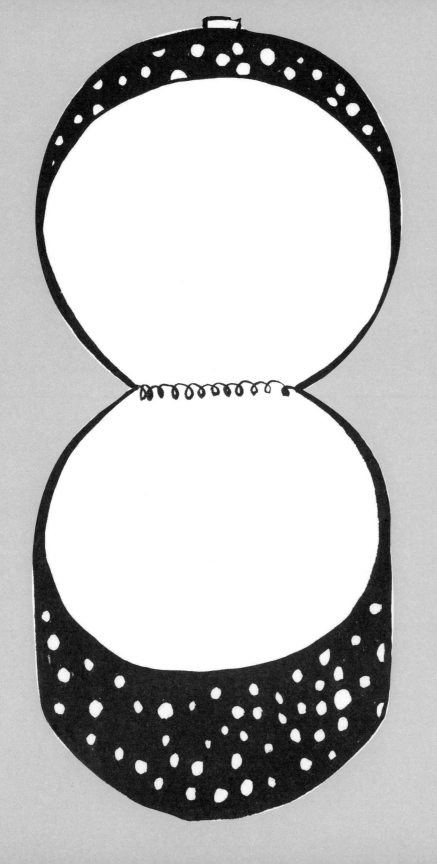

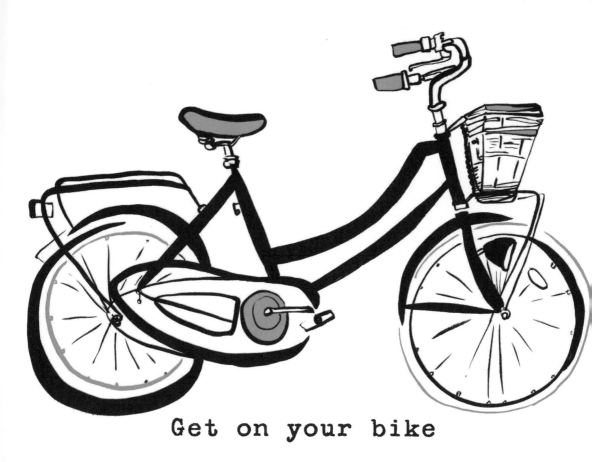

Get on your bike

How many times have you driven the car this week?
Taken the bus? The train?

Get around under your own steam as much as you can
this week. Walk, ride (wear a helmet, even if it
ruins your hairstyle), even run if you can.

If you can't do it the whole way, then just do
it some of the way. Allow yourself the time to
increase your activity.

Monday

Tuesday

Wednesday

Thursday

Friday

What did you eat today?

WEEK
16

Saturday

Sunday

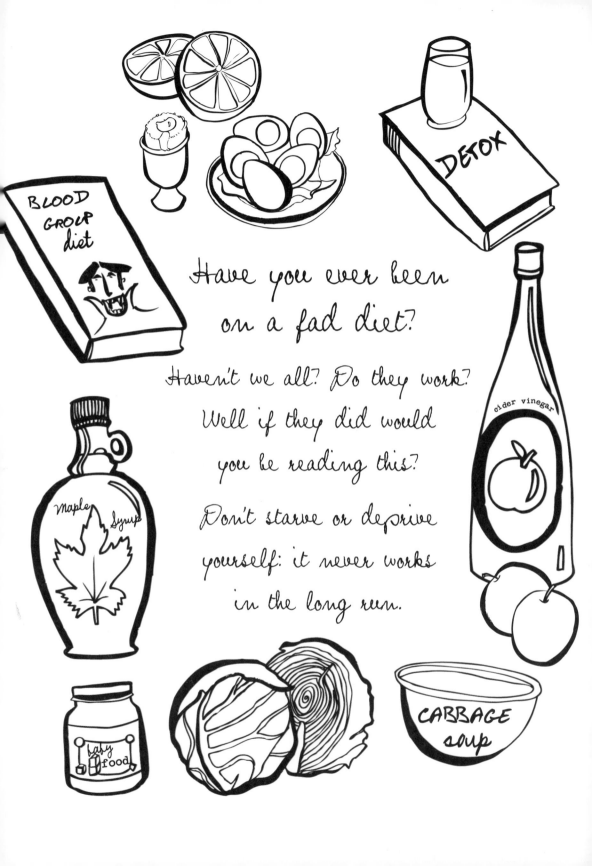

Have you ever been
on a fad diet?

Haven't we all? Do they work?
Well if they did would
you be reading this?

Don't starve or deprive
yourself: it never works
in the long run.

Log your fitness progress

WEEK 16

Monday

Tuesday

Wednesday

Thursday

Friday

THE weigh-IN

WEIGHT : ———
WAIST : ———
HEART
RATE : ———

Saturday

Sunday

my new recipes

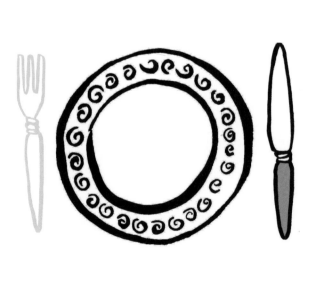

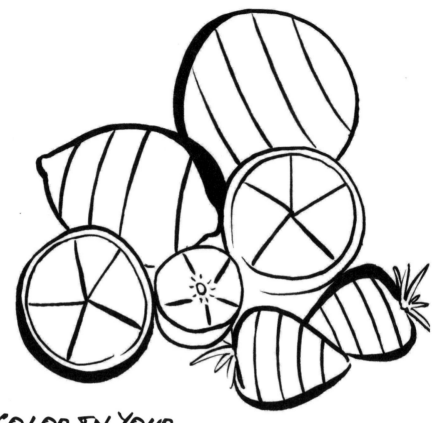

COLOR IN YOUR FRUIT SERVINGS EACH DAY

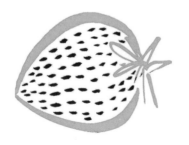

Shade a segment of one of these fruits—one fruit for each day this week—when you've eaten one of your portions of fruits or vegetables.

Monday

Tuesday

Wednesday

Thursday

Friday

What did
you eat
today?

Saturday

Sunday

WEEK
17

Challenge: how many times can you get active this week?

make this a week when you don't sit still!

Shade a segment of the bicycle every time you do some kind of activity for a few minutes at a time, even a little walk, or some housework, or taking the stairs instead of the elevator.

Fill in the whole bike!

Don't forget to stretch and to rest after strenuous exercise.

 strenuous

medium

 light

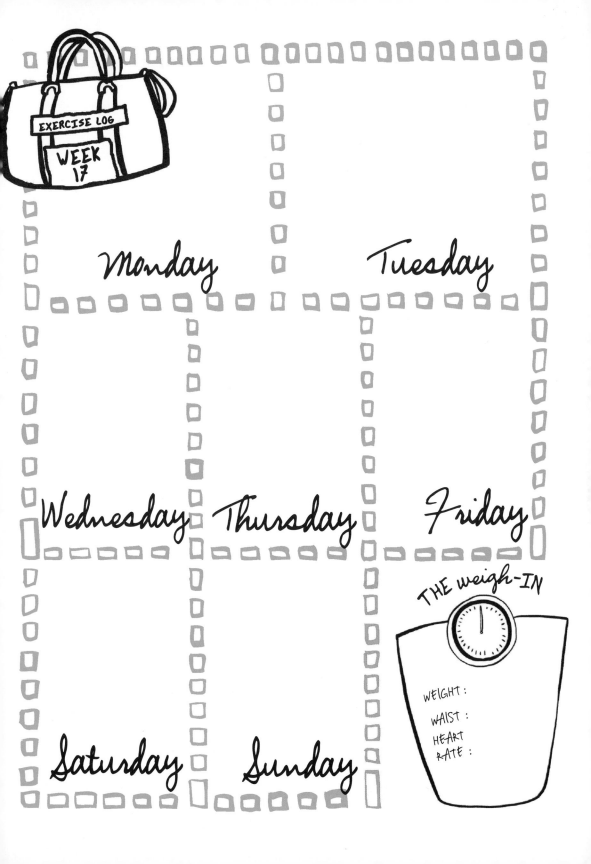

EXERCISE LOG
WEEK 17

Monday

Tuesday

Wednesday

Thursday

Friday

THE weigh-IN

WEIGHT :

WAIST :

HEART
RATE :

Saturday

Sunday

Monday

Tuesday

Wednesday

Thursday

Friday

What did
you eat
today?

Saturday

Sunday

WEEK
18

your real friends are your cheerleaders

GO TEAM TORTOISE

Exercise Log

WEEK 18

Monday

Tuesday

Wednesday

Thursday

Friday

Sunday

THE weigh-IN

WEIGHT :

WAIST :

HEART
RATE :

Saturday

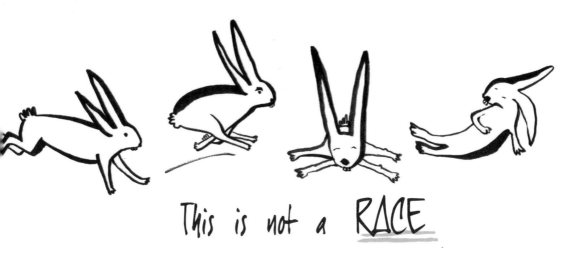

This is not a RACE

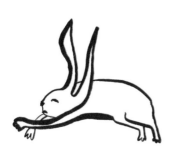

Slow

and

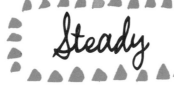

Steady

will get you there!

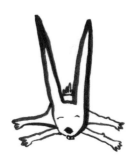

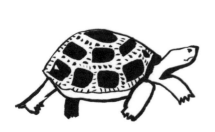
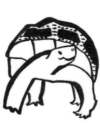
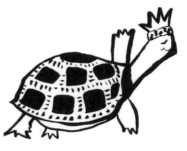

Don't become a diet drag ...

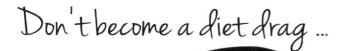

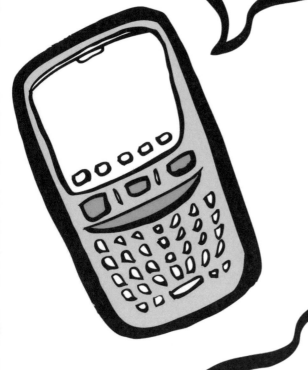

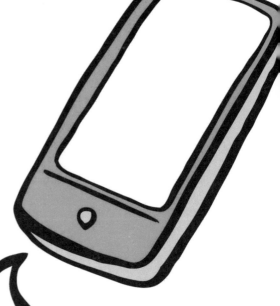

Monday

Tuesday

Wednesday

Thursday

Friday

Saturday

Sunday

WEEK 19

Monday

Tuesday

Wednesday

Thursday

Friday

Saturday

Sunday

THE weigh-IN

WEIGHT :

WAIST :

HEART RATE :

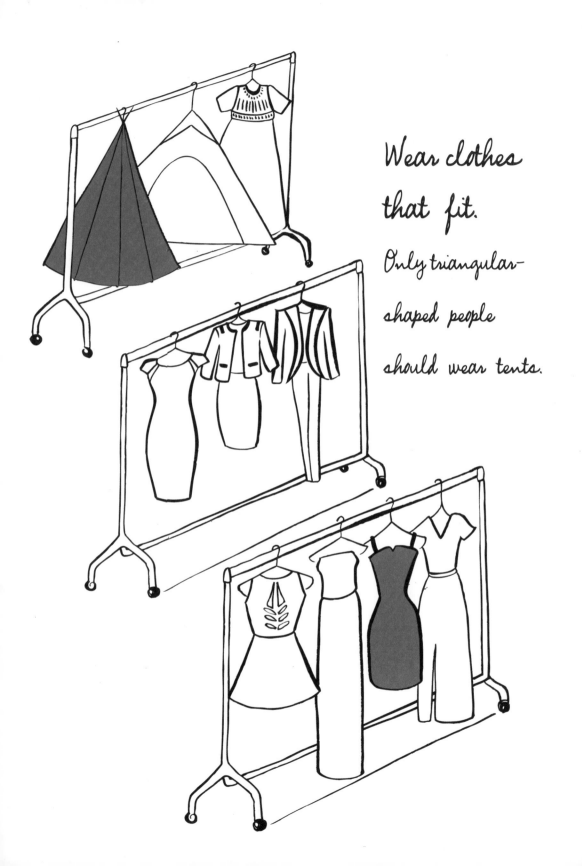

Wear clothes
that fit.
Only triangular-
shaped people
should wear tents.

"NOTHING IS

IMPOSSIBLE.

THE WORD ITSELF SAYS

'I'm possible!'"

—AUDREY HEPBURN

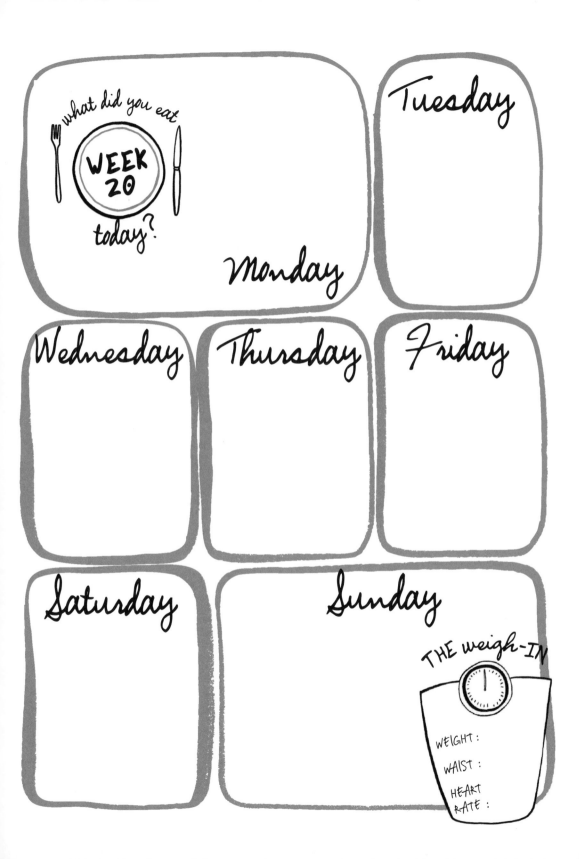

what did you eat

WEEK 20

today?

Monday

Tuesday

Wednesday

Thursday

Friday

Saturday

Sunday

THE weigh-IN

WEIGHT :

WAIST :

HEART
RATE :

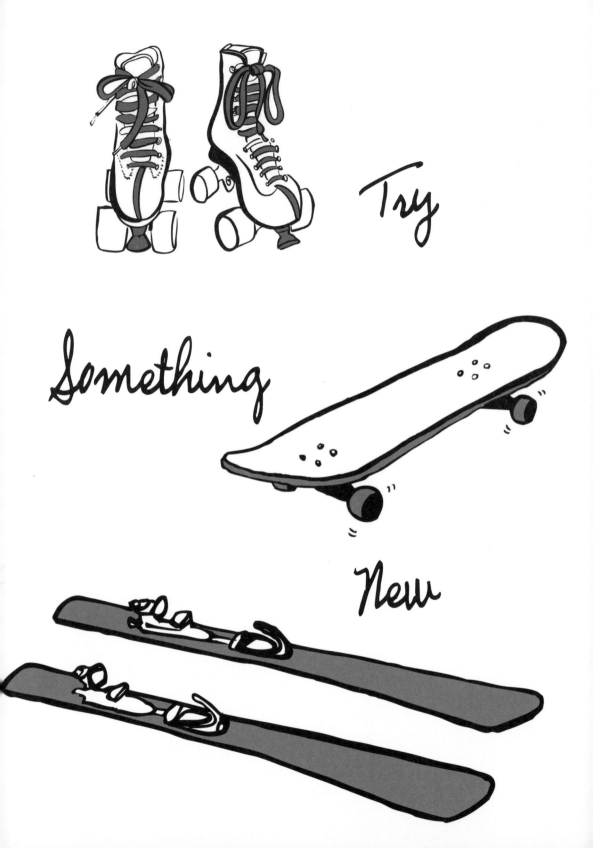

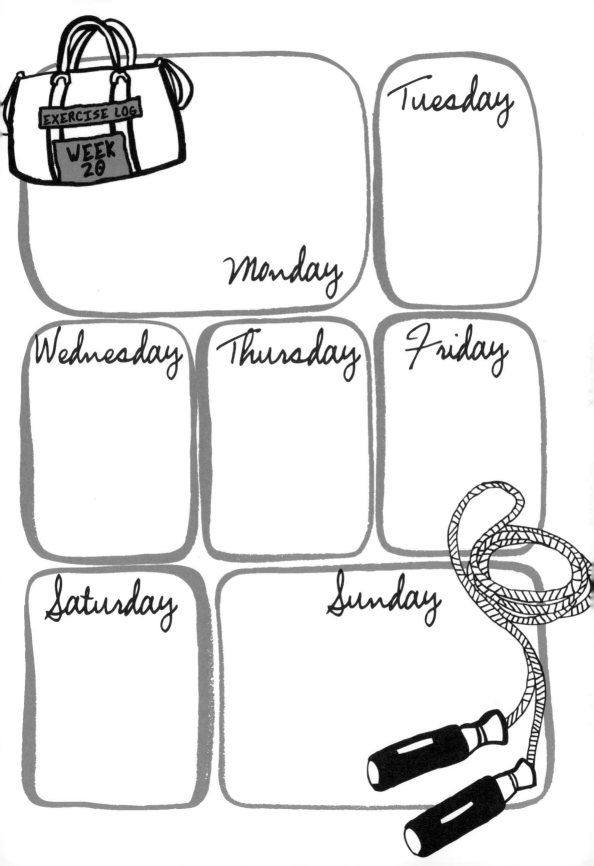

EXERCISE LOG
WEEK 20

Monday

Tuesday

Wednesday

Thursday

Friday

Saturday

Sunday

an apple a day . . .

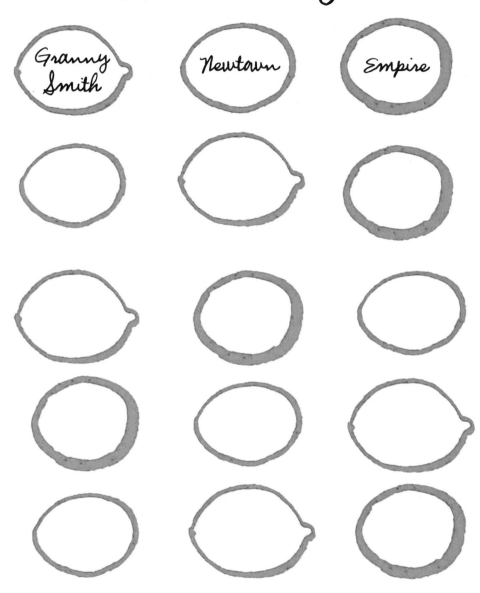

Granny Smith

Newtown

Empire

Fill out your five fruits a day, as you
have them, on this page.

Food diary
WEEK 21

Monday

Tuesday

Wednesday

Thursday

Friday

Saturday

Sunday

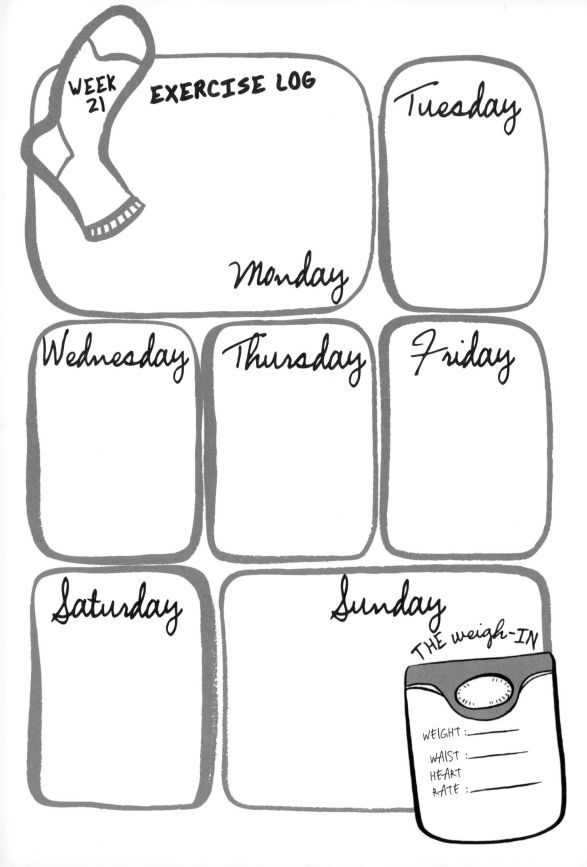

WEEK 21

EXERCISE LOG

Tuesday

Monday

Wednesday

Thursday

Friday

Saturday

Sunday

THE weigh-IN

WEIGHT :_____
WAIST :_____
HEART
RATE :_____

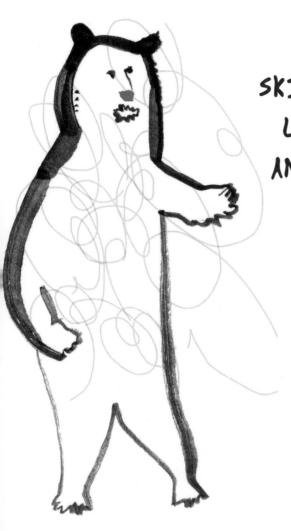

SKIPPING MEALS WILL
LEAVE YOU HUNGRY
AND FEELING LIKE A
GRIZZLY BEAR!

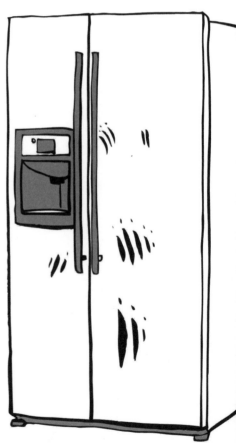

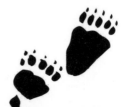

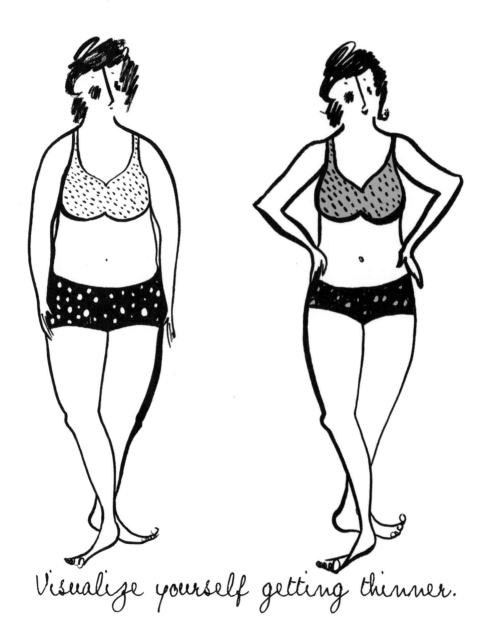

Visualize yourself getting thinner.

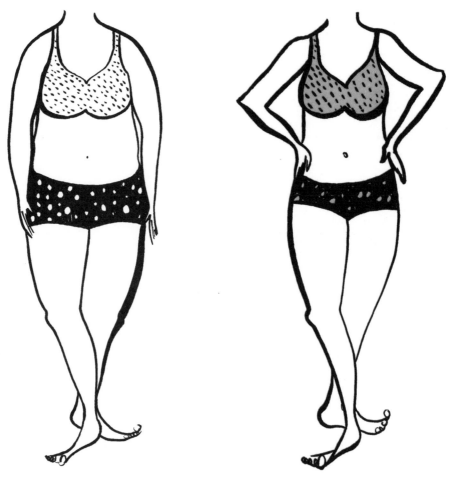

Draw yourself getting thinner.

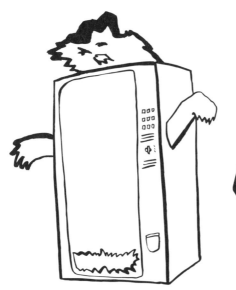

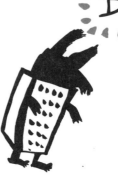

DANGER

DANGER

Keep Healthy
Snacks
at Work

...or you might be
at the mercy of

THE VENDING
MACHINE!

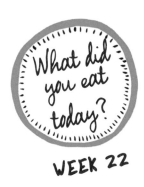

What did you eat today?

WEEK 22

Monday

Tuesday

Wednesday

Thursday

Friday

Saturday

Sunday

THE weigh-IN

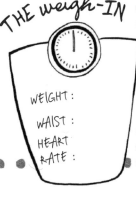

WEIGHT :

WAIST :

HEART RATE :

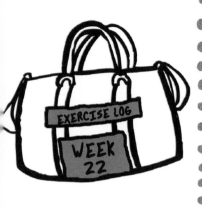

EXERCISE LOG

WEEK 22

Monday

Tuesday

Wednesday

Thursday

Friday

Saturday

Sunday

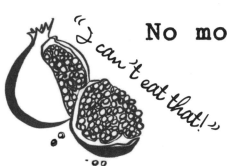

No more excuses...

Write your negative
thoughts on this page.
Turn the page and decide
that is the end of them.

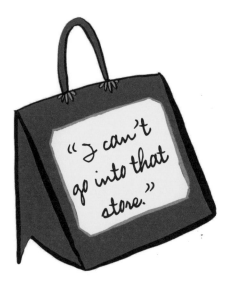

"I can't
go into that
store."

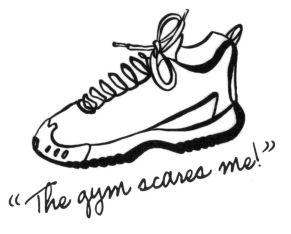

"The gym scares me!"

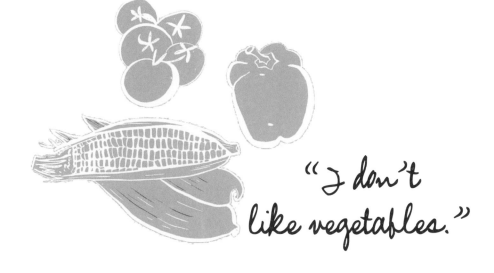

"I don't
like vegetables."

Monday

Tuesday

Wednesday

Thursday

Friday

what did you eat

WEEK
23

today?

Saturday

Sunday

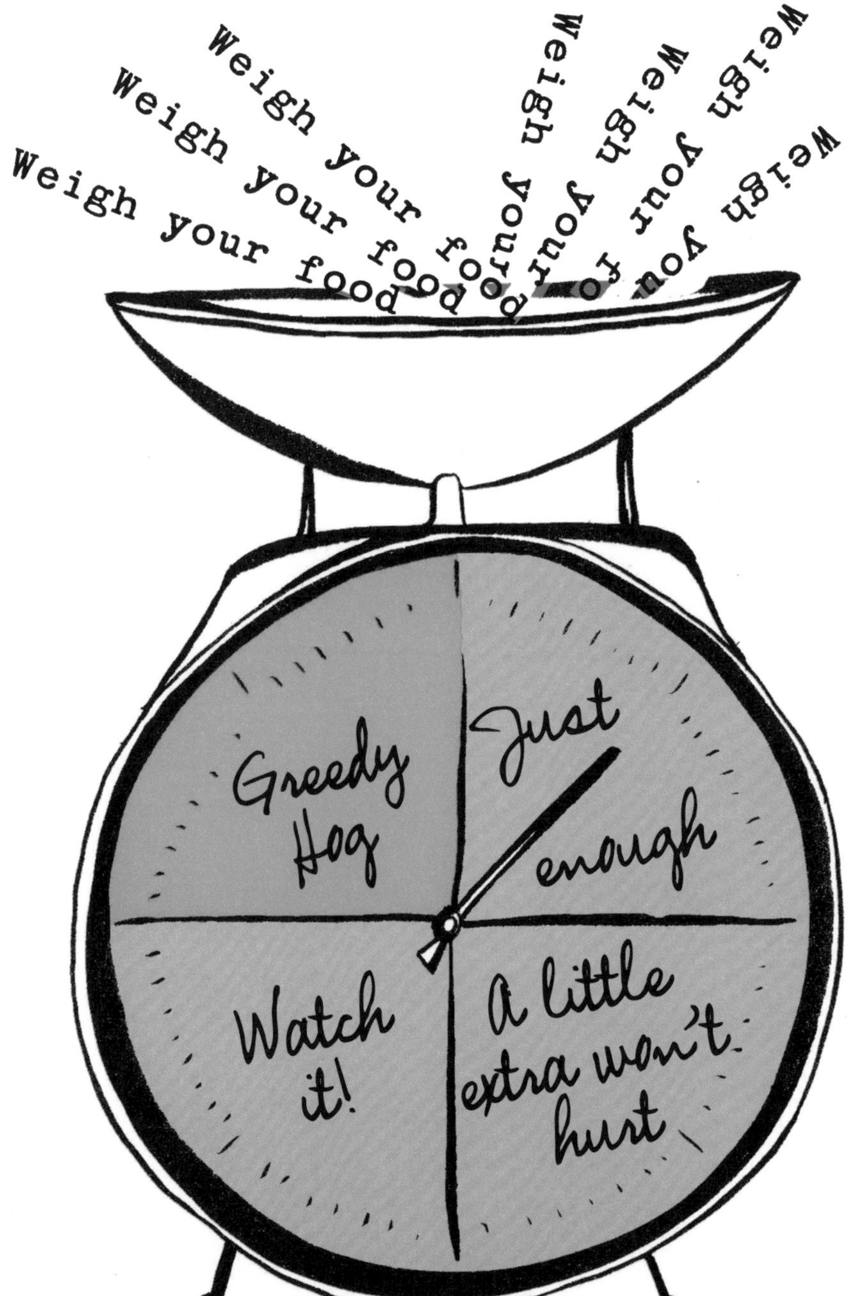
Weigh your food
Weigh your food
Weigh your food
Weigh your food
Weigh your food
Weigh your food
Weigh your food
Greedy Hog
Just enough
Watch it!
A little extra won't hurt

WEEK 23
EXERCISE LOG

Monday

Tuesday

Wednesday

Thursday

Friday

Saturday

Sunday

THE weigh-IN

WEIGHT : _____

WAIST : _____
HEART
RATE : _____

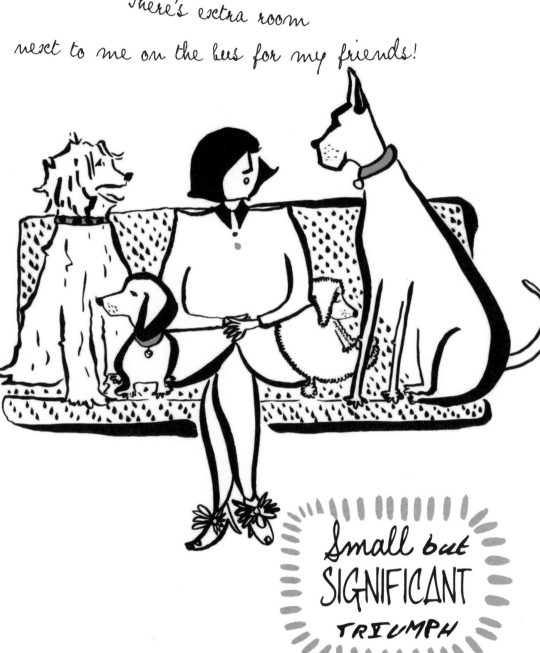

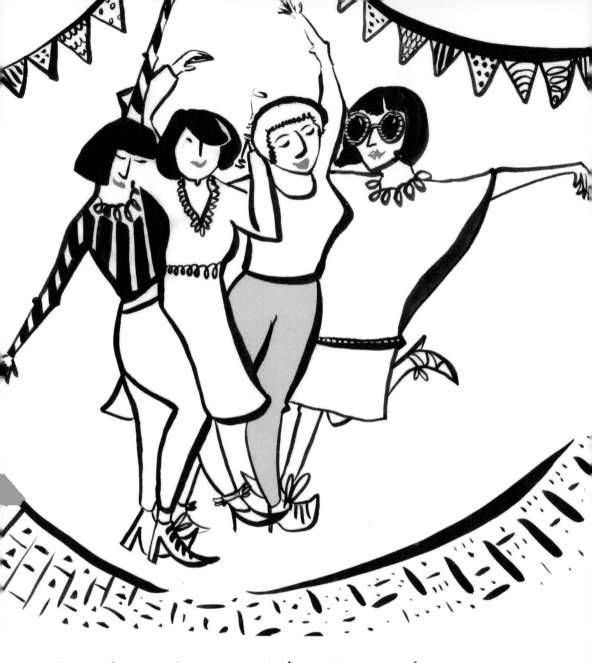

Dancing like an idiot is good exercise. Don't avoid nights out because you are "on a diet." Plan! And make good choices.

Monday

Tuesday

Wednesday

Thursday

Friday

Saturday

Sunday

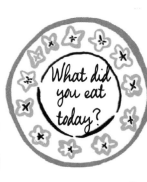

What did you eat today?

WEEK 24

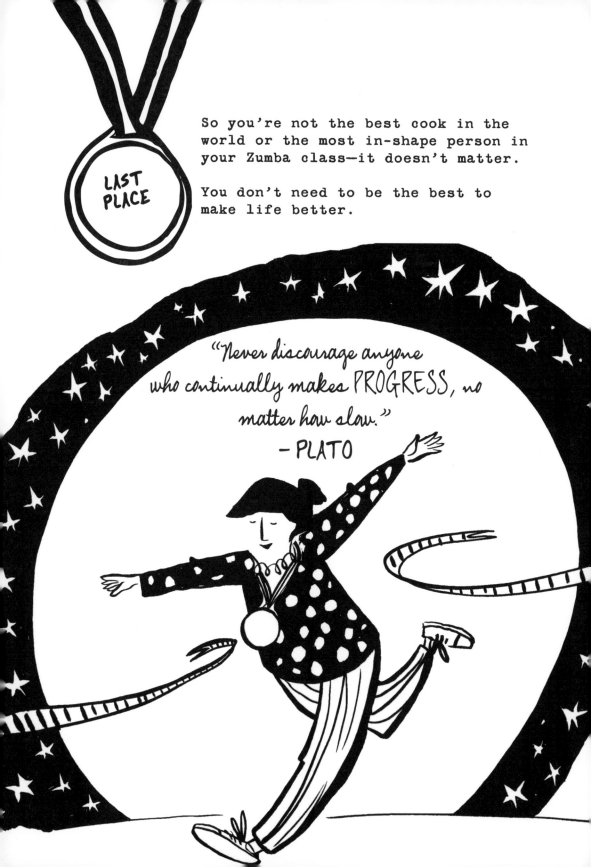

So you're not the best cook in the world or the most in-shape person in your Zumba class—it doesn't matter.

You don't need to be the best to make life better.

LAST PLACE

"Never discourage anyone who continually makes PROGRESS, no matter how slow."
— PLATO

Monday

EXERCISE LOG
WEEK 24

Tuesday

Wednesday

Thursday

Friday

Saturday

Sunday

THE weigh-IN

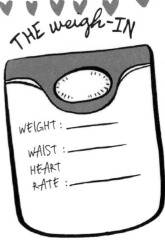

WEIGHT : _____

WAIST : _____

HEART
RATE : _____

Monday

Tuesday

Wednesday

Thursday

Friday

Saturday

Sunday

What did you eat today?

WEEK 25

WEEK 25

Monday

Tuesday

Wednesday

Thursday

Friday

Saturday

Sunday

THE
Weigh
IN

WEIGHT : _____

WAIST : _____

HEART
RATE : _____

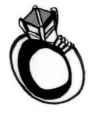

"My wedding band fits again."

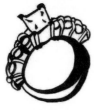

What's your

Small but SIGNIFICANT TRIUMPH

this week?

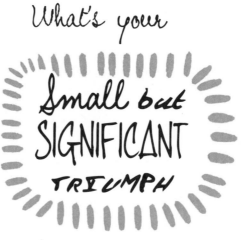

What did you eat today?

WEEK 26

Monday

Tuesday

Wednesday

Thursday

Friday

Saturday

Sunday

THE weigh-IN

WEIGHT :

WAIST :

HEART RATE :

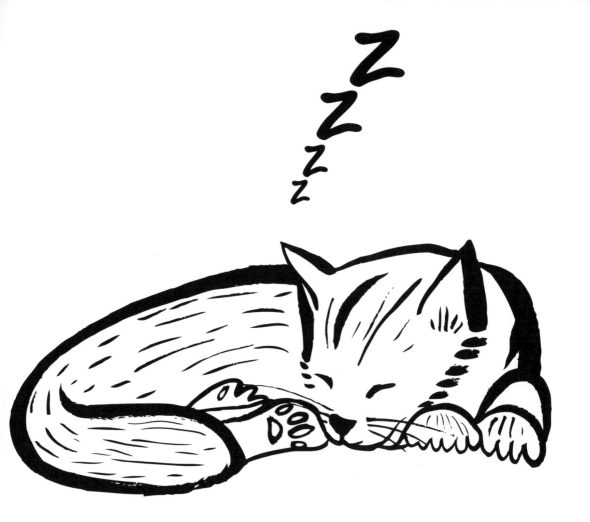

Get enough sleep!
Sleep helps you cope with most
things, including healthy eating.

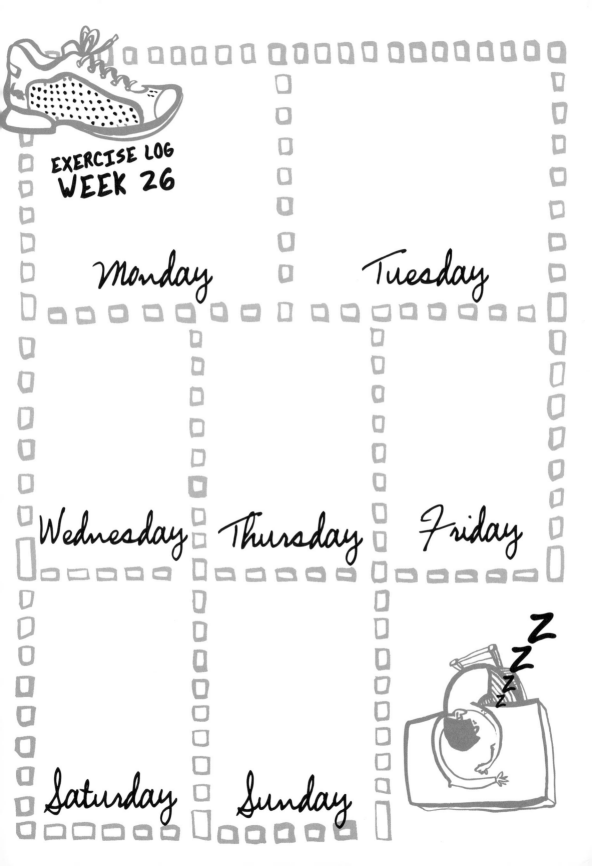

EXERCISE LOG
WEEK 26

Monday

Tuesday

Wednesday

Thursday

Friday

Saturday

Sunday

My New Recipes

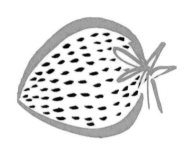

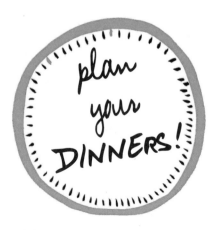

plan your DINNERS!

EAT

FROM

SMALLER

dishes.

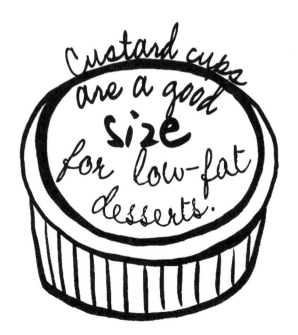

Custard cups are a good size for low-fat desserts.

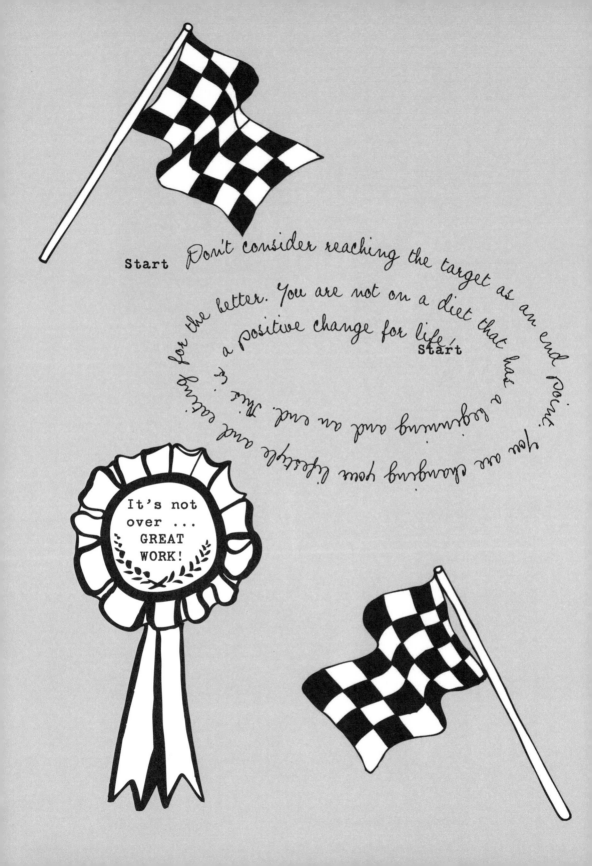

Start

Don't consider reaching the target as an end point. You are not on a diet that has a beginning and an end. That is a positive change for life.

Start

You are changing your lifestyle and eating for the better.

It's not over ... GREAT WORK!

Monday

Tuesday

Wednesday

Thursday

Friday

What did you eat today?

WEEK 27

Saturday

Sunday

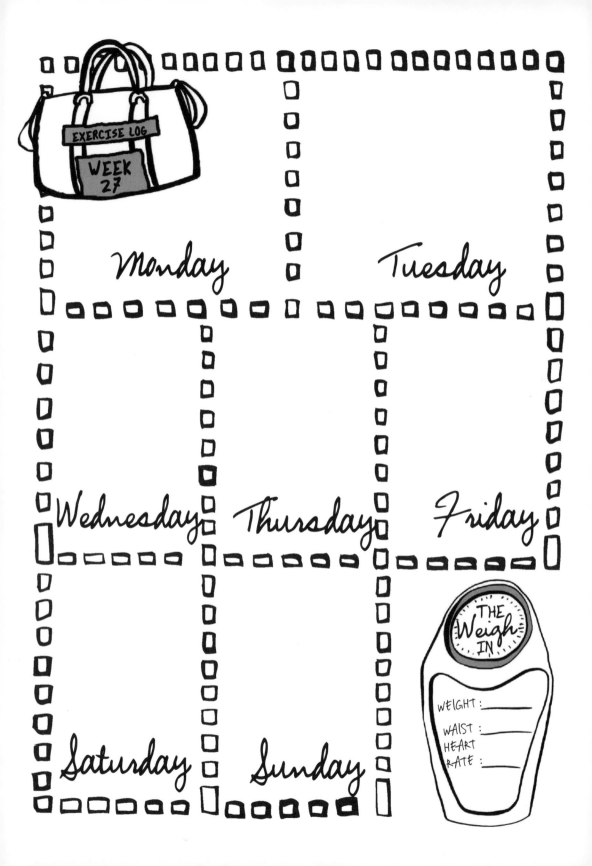

EXERCISE LOG

WEEK 27

Monday

Tuesday

Wednesday

Thursday

Friday

Saturday

Sunday

THE Weigh IN

WEIGHT : _____

WAIST : _____

HEART
RATE : _____

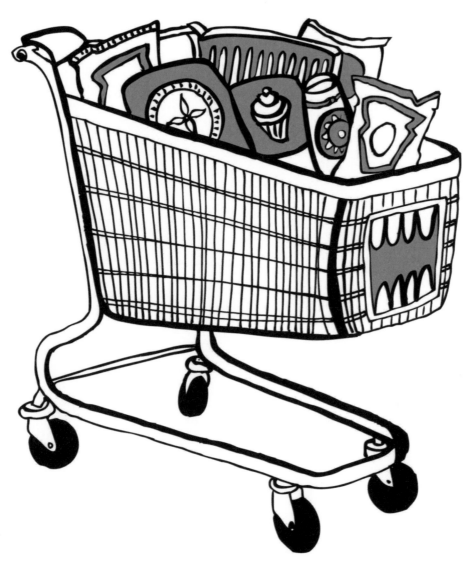

A hungry feeling is not a good shopping companion.

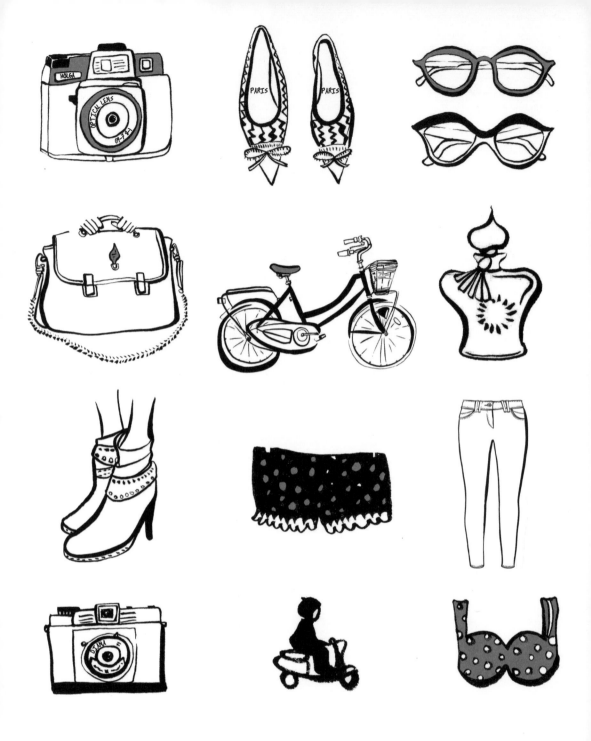

Reward yourself

What did you eat today?

WEEK 29

Monday

Tuesday

Wednesday

Thursday

Friday

Saturday

Sunday

How do you feel now?

Choose descriptive words and write them in the thought bubbles.

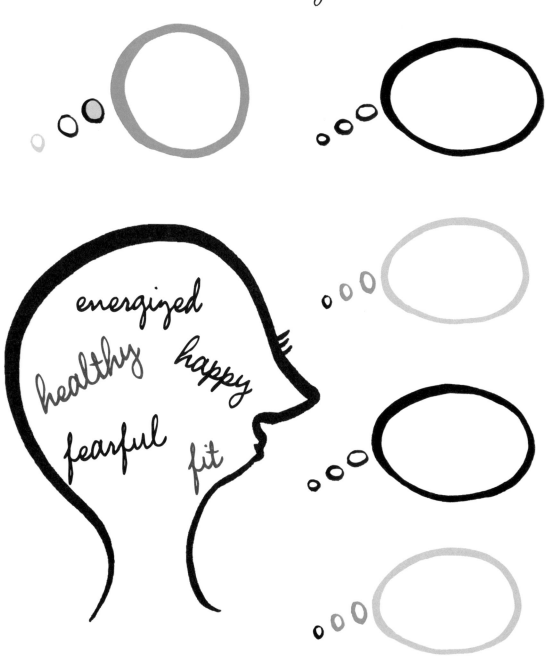

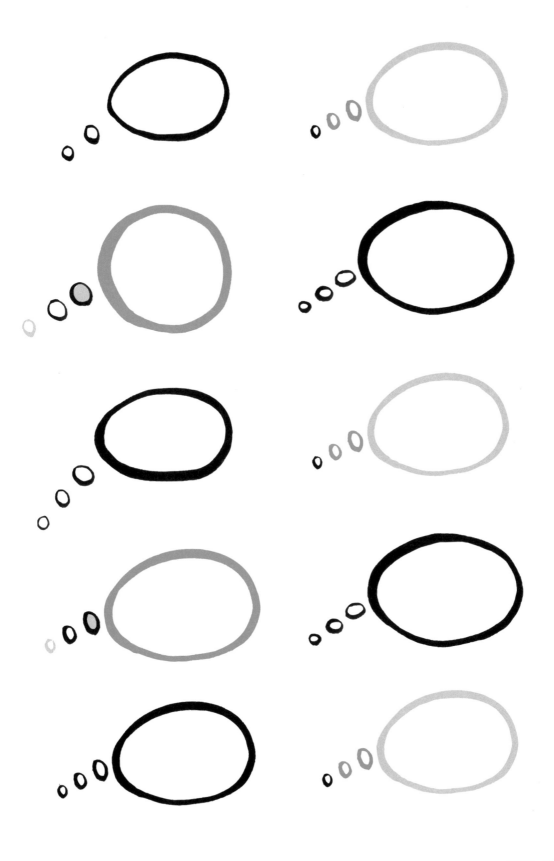

How far are you now from
your target weight?
Draw it on the scale.

It doesn't matter how far
you've come as long as
you are still
making PROGRESS.

Record your

measurements now:

Neck

. . . .

Chest

. . . .

Waist

. . . .

Upper arm

. . . .

Wrist

. . . .

Thigh

. . . .

Calf

. . . .

Ankle

. . . .

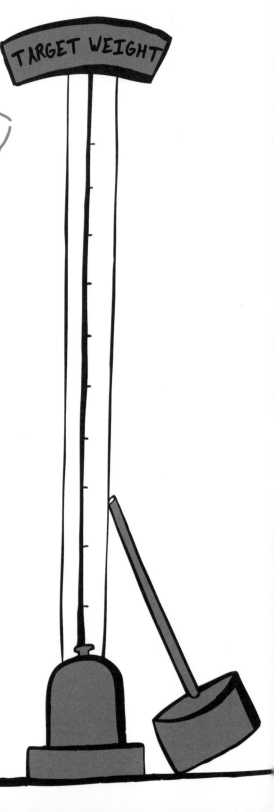

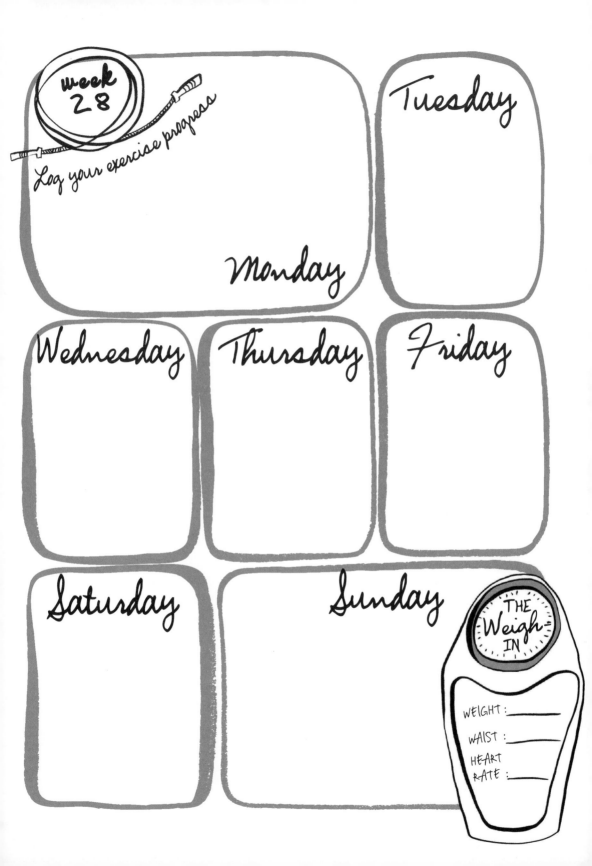

week 28

Log your exercise progress

Monday

Tuesday

Wednesday

Thursday

Friday

Saturday

Sunday

THE Weigh IN

WEIGHT : _____

WAIST : _____

HEART RATE : _____

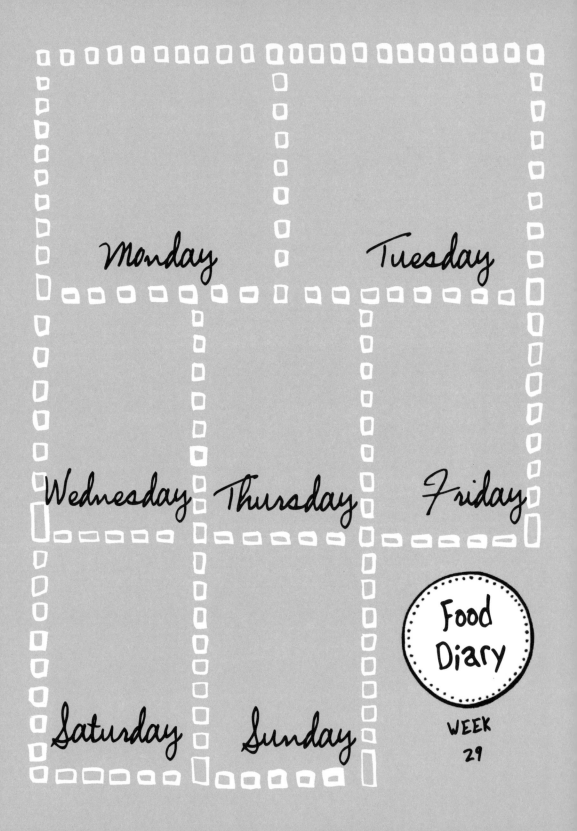

Monday

Tuesday

Wednesday

Thursday

Friday

Food Diary

WEEK 29

Saturday

Sunday